Distinctive Feature Analysis of Misarticulations

DISTINCTIVE FEATURE ANALYSIS OF MISARTICULATIONS

Leija V. McReynolds, Ph.D.
Professor
Hearing and Speech Department
University of Kansas Medical Center;
Research Associate
Bureau of Child Research
University of Kansas

Deedra L. Engmann, M.A.
Assistant Director and Research Associate
Speech and Language Research Laboratory
Kansas Center for Mental Retardation and Human Development
University of Kansas Medical Center

University Park Press
Baltimore · London · Tokyo

UNIVERSITY PARK PRESS
International Publishers in Science and Medicine
233 East Redwood Street
Baltimore, Maryland 21202

Typeset by The Composing Room of Michigan
Printed in the United States of America
Second printing, February 1977
Third printing, September 1978

Library of Congress Cataloging in Publication Data

McReynolds, Leija V
Distinctive feature analysis of misarticulations.

Bibliography: p.
Includes index.
1. Articulation disorders. 2. Distinctive features (Linguistics) 3. Speech disorders in children.
I. Engmann, Deedra L., joint author. II. Title.
[DNLM: 1. Speech therapy. WM475 M174d]
RJ496.S7M3 618.9'28'552 75-8963
ISBN 0-8391-0755-2

Contents

Preface

Viewing misarticulations as distinctive feature errors requires application of linguistic theory and methodology. Thus, procedures for completing a distinctive feature analysis are somewhat different from conventional articulation evaluation procedures. The purpose of this book is twofold: (1) to instruct speech pathologists to conduct a distinctive feature analysis of a child's misarticulations, and (2) to demonstrate how information derived from the analysis can be used to develop systematic articulation training programs. Although distinctive feature theory is discussed, emphasis is placed on application of the theory to children's articulation problems. The text is not a general articulation text; the content is limited to application of feature analysis for evaluation and treatment of articulation errors. Other approaches are not described. The authors, however, recognize that a great deal of useful information is available from other areas of research in articulation and speech. Speech pathologists are encouraged to use this information to supplement the distinctive feature analysis or, when appropriate, to use information from the distinctive feature analysis to supplement other approaches to articulation evaluation and treatment.

Acknowledgments

The authors wish to thank the people who were research assistants during the time when the research reported in this book was being conducted: Kay Huston, Shannon Bennett, Judith Branch, Thomas Booth, Joan Kohn, and Gail Williams. The research was supported by Research Grant HD 00870 from the National Institute of Child Health and Human Development, and Research Grant NS 10468 from the National Institute of Neurological Diseases and Stroke to the Bureau of Child Research at the University of Kansas.

For their help in conducting distinctive feature workshops we would like to acknowledge Lois Huffman and Gary Holdgrafer. We would especially like to thank Mary Elbert, Kenneth Ruder, and Ralph Shelton for their useful comments and advice during the writing of the manuscript. Several people helped type the manuscript, and we wish to thank Melanie Faust, Lori Jantz, and Joan Harvey for taking their turns.

Introduction

The focus of this book is on the application of distinctive theory to an understanding of children's misarticulations, and on the development of a distinctive feature analysis to correct these misarticulations. Theoretical background is covered only to the extent that it explains the principles inherent in distinctive feature theory. The principles serve as guidelines for designing and conducting articulation treatment programs.

Part I provides background for understanding the principles involved in distinctive feature theory as it was developed by linguists. Chomsky and Halle's distinctive feature system, the system used in this book, is discussed in relation to other feature systems. Part I also explains application of distinctive feature theory to articulation problems. Information from research exploring the relevance of distinctive features to children's articulation errors is presented. A rationale for applying a distinctive feature analysis to articulation errors is discussed in relation to the theory and the research.

Programmed instruction for completing a distinctive feature analysis is found in Part II. This part presents the step-by-step procedures used in a distinctive feature analysis. Responses on an articulation test by two children are used in teaching the procedures. Each step is followed by exercises.

Data from the distinctive feature analysis in Part II are used in Part III to develop articulation training programs for the two sample children from Part II. The third part provides principles for designing distinctive feature training procedures. As in Part II, exercises provide practice on the procedures necessary for designing training programs.

I

DISTINCTIVE FEATURE THEORY

In this part an attempt is made to explain the relevance of distinctive features to articulation problems. An introduction to distinctive feature theory, sufficient for describing the relationship between features and articulation, is offered. The feature system used in the present analysis is explained so as to place it into perspective with current theory and research in distinctive features. Finally, a distinctive feature approach for evaluating articulation errors and developing articulation remediation programs is compared briefly to more conventional approaches to articulation problems.

1

Introduction to Distinctive Feature Theory

Linguists describe how children acquire the phonology of their language and discover the universal elements of languages (Chomsky and Halle, 1968; Jakobson, Fant, and Halle, 1952; Jakobson and Halle, 1956; Postal, 1968; Saporta, 1955). They are interested in developing a phonological theory that will describe the basic articulatory and sound elements of languages, and the rules that relate them to meaning. Phonological theory describes how children acquire the phonemes of their culture.

On the basis of information derived from descriptive data, linguists formulate theoretical propositions to explain the linguistic structures of languages and how they are acquired. In an effort to find the universal, discrete components of language, Jakobson, Fant, and Halle (1952) made articulatory, acoustical, and perceptual measurements of speech. Results of measurements on these three levels led them to propose that phonemes are not the fundamental elements of language, but that there are elements called distinctive features which are basic to phonemes. According to Berko and Brown (1960, pp. 525–526), "the 'distinctive features' of an individual phoneme would be those aspects of the process of articulation and their acoustic consequences that serve to contrast one phoneme from another."

The distinctive features of Jakobson, Fant, and Halle were proposed as universal features in that they were not language-specific. Rather, they were articulatory elements generated by speakers of all languages; that is, these were features learned by all children, and were language-independent. The universal features were defined in binary terms. A feature was either present (+) or absent (−) in a phoneme. In any language, the features serve to distinguish phonemes from each other, and therefore are linguistically relevant. When two phonemes differ from each other only in one feature, that feature is linguistically relevant since it functions to differentiate two phonemes in a language. According to the theory, an individual who has acquired all the features has acquired the elements which would enable him to learn the phonemes of his language. Jakobson, Fant, and Halle's original distinctive features were based on phonemics. Accordingly, they were not particularly concerned whether the features were integrated into a system that included other aspects of grammar, such as syntax and semantics.

Recently, speech scientists and others

engaged in delineating the physical and acoustical attributes of phonemes in speech have questioned the relationship of distinctive features to speech and language (Delattre, 1968; Liberman, Cooper, Shankweiler and Studdert-Kennedy, 1967; MacNeilage, 1970; Peterson and Shoup, 1966; Singh and Black, 1966). In the course of extensive research in speech perception and production, investigators have accumulated much information about these attributes. Their data led them to question the psychological reality of the distinctive features and their binary nature. In addition, concern was expressed as to whether the proposed features were the appropriate ones.

Researchers and theorists alike recognize that features, like phonemes, are abstractions. They are idealized forms which are not realized in actual utterances by speakers of a language (Fant, 1971; Singh, 1971; Wilson, 1966). There is not a one-to-one correspondence between the physical production of a feature and its description. The articulating organs do not attain their target configuration in speech. The relationship is one of "allophones" and "phones" to phonemes in which the target sound is the phoneme. When an individual produces a sound, the physical production does not conform precisely to the somewhat static articulatory description of the model. This variation from a phoneme may be an allophone, and each production is called a phone.

Several variables account for the differences between a phoneme and its production by a speaker. Among these are the different contexts and environments in which a sound is produced, and physiological differences among persons producing phonemes. Likewise, changes in the individual as he produces the same sound on different occasions and the conditions under which the same sound is produced in successive articulations influence phonemic production.

Some variations are predictable. For example, allophones consist of productions that are recognized and accepted by listeners as predictable variations within a specific phoneme class. For instance, English speakers accept the [t] in *stop* and *top* as the /t/ phoneme although it is aspirated in one context and unaspirated in the other. The two productions are allophones of the /t/ phoneme.

Some variations cannot be predicted because all of the variables acting upon a production cannot be predicted. The characteristics composing the variations may be different each time an individual produces a phoneme. An individual production of a phoneme is called a "phone." For example, the [l] in the word "love" in three successive repetitions by one person is different in each utterance. Only some variables responsible for the variations can be specified. Some cannot be identified at the moment of production, although they also operate to make each phone (each repetition) different from the others. Thus, each time a particular sound is produced, the single production of the phoneme is identified as a phone.

Because no two productions are the same, the physical and acoustical characteristics of phonemes in utterances do not match the characteristics of the target phonemes, as they are described in discrete terms. The attributes of a phoneme, when produced by a speaker, are actually at some point on a continuum in terms of the specifics used to describe the target. More precisely, because of the variables influencing the actual production, a feature is probably never entirely present or absent. Investigators, speech scientists in particular, suggest that an accurate description of a phoneme production would detail the variations. That is, the physical and acoustical characteristics composing actual productions would be specified. Speech scientists are less concerned with the development of formal linguistic theory (defining the universal features) than are linguists. Often they are empiricists conducting extensive experimental work directed at defining the physical, acoustical, and perceptual attributes of phonemes.

Some attributes correspond to the distinctive features proposed by linguists. On the other hand, noticeable discrepancies have been found between some articulatory features proposed by linguists and the perceptual (and, by extrapolation, physiological) configurations occurring during production of phonemes by speakers of English. A few individuals have proposed sets of features based on their perceptual experimental studies (Graham and House, 1971; Miller and Nicely, 1955; Peters, 1963; Singh and Becker, 1972; Singh, Woods, and Becker, 1972; Wickelgren, 1966).

Most of these systems contain linguistically relevant features and other features which are not linguistically relevant. The features, therefore, may be described as phonemic and phonetic. They are rather precise descriptions of phoneme attributes as produced by English speakers. A full phonetic transcription of an utterance, then, would specify values for all features on a scale which corresponds to the physical productions. This detailed feature specification and description is different from the binary specification of distinctive features as proposed by linguists. For linguists, such specification is not appropriate to formal linguistic theory.

Yet, linguists too, are concerned about the relationship between universal features and articulatory attributes present in utterances of phonemes. Since their interest is directed toward developing linguistic theory, however, identification of all the features, all the physical properties of each phoneme production, is not pertinent. In principle, such detailed descriptions would defeat the concept of distinctive features because features would then become language-specific instead of language-independent. As such, they would not be universal. Clearly, in this capacity they would not contribute significantly to a general theory of language.

Some linguists point out the distinction between features that form contrasts in a language, and features that do not function in that manner. Specifically, features may be categorized as distinctive or nondistinctive (Cairns and Williams, 1973). When the features in a sound produced by a speaker do not serve to contrast phonemes, they belong to the nondistinctive feature category and are considered redundant. On the other hand, when the articulatory configurations are found in several languages and serve to contrast phonemes, they are classified as universal (distinctive) features. It is these distinctive features which contribute to the formation of general linguistic theory.

It is possible to specify both the distinctive and nondistinctive features in the actual production of a sound. When only the distinctive features are specified, the bundle of features compose a unit, or segment, known as a phoneme, and the description is a phonological representation. When both distinctive and nondistinctive features are employed in the description, it is a phonetic representation limited to a phone. Phonological rules function to relate the two representations. Knowledge of these rules enables the speaker-hearer to derive the underlying phonological representation from the phonetic one. In developing phonological theory, linguists specify the rules which relate the phonological and phonetic levels.

2

Chomsky and Halle's Distinctive Feature Theory

A somewhat different theory of distinctive features has been proposed by Chomsky and Halle (1968). It departs from other theories because it does not regard the phoneme as an autonomous unit; instead, it is concerned with a theory of generative grammar. A set of distinctive features, derived from phonemes as individual structures, is not considered in a generative model. Within this theory, distinctive features are defined in the context of syntactic components. Phonological components cannot be treated independently of syntax, since phonetic variations occur as a function of syntactic rules. Indeed, a theory of generative phonology requires that phonetic variations be somewhat dependent upon syntax.

Although phonemes are involved, their theory is not derived from the phonemes of any specific language. Rather, it is based on the sounds of languages in general. From their study of the structure of linguistic systems, Chomsky and Halle identified the phonetic properties that characterize the utterances of several languages and can be controlled in speech. These properties form the set of distinctive features they propose as basic articulatory features in all languages.

The features are independent of the grammar of any particular language. A feature, or parameter, that is never significant in any language is not a feature, distinctive or nondistinctive; i.e., if an articulatory parameter does not function linguistically in any language, it is not a feature at all. Only features that are significant in natural languages are included in the Chomsky-Halle conception of distinctive features.

This limitation is useful for linguistic theory because it restricts the set of permissible features. In contrast, a theory based on phonemes in which any vocal dimension man produces can be a permissible feature is less manageable because of the vast number of possible features. Chomsky and Halle suggest that the features in their theory represent the phonetic capabilities of man. Consequently, they are the same for all languages. Because their features are derived from languages in general, rather than from a particular language, they need not concern themselves with accounting for the presence of nondistinctive features. In fact, the concept of nondistinctive features is irrelevant in their theory.

Although Chomsky and Halle see no need to separate features into two classes, they agree that the differences between the idealized distinctive features and their actual form in utterances need to be recognized within the context of a theory of language. They explain the lack of a one-to-one relationship between the phonological form and its phonetic representation by suggesting that features have two functions. Instead of dividing features into distinctive and nondistinctive classes, Chomsky and Halle propose that all distinctive features may operate on two levels. The authors distinguish between distinctive features functioning on a classificatory level and distinctive features operating on a phonetic level.

When distinctive features operate on a classificatory level, they provide feature categories that are significant for any specific language. At this level, the values for features that are significant in any given language are noted. In their classificatory capacity features are binary; they specify whether the segment (the consonant or vowel in an utterance) is within a feature category. Thus, a segment may be classified as a member of a feature category, or as not a member of a feature category. For example, the sound may be a member of the feature category *continuancy,* in which case it is plus (+) for that feature. If it is not a member of that category, it is minus (−) for that feature. In this dichotomy, sounds are either in or out of a feature category and are specified as either present or absent in a sound. There are no in-between specifications.

On the phonetic level, features function as properties. Features on the phonetic level are the same predetermined features as those in the classificatory level. At the phonetic level, however, features that may be significant in any language are designated. That is, if an articulatory property is significant for several languages, the property is a phonetic feature. This does not mean, necessarily, that the feature is significant for the particular language in which the utterance is recorded. It is present in the production of the sound, and a full description of the sound would include specification of the degree to which that feature is present. In their phonetic function, features receive a physical interpretation. Instead of a binary specification, the description is multivalued on a physical and acoustical continuum. In particular, the degree to which a segment is characterized by the feature is specified. For example, a sound may be described as "noncontinuant" and "moderately aspirated" on the phonetic feature level. At this level, contextual variables are taken into account.

To show these two functions, Chomsky and Halle use the conventional slash marks (/ /) used to enclose phonemes, and square brackets ([ ]) commonly used to enclose phones. When features function as classificatory devices, they use the diagonals; when features function phonetically, they use square brackets. Some features which man is capable of producing are not significant in any language; these articulatory parameters are not distinctive features. They would not function as either phonetic or classificatory features.

It is not unusual for the classificatory and phonetic level descriptions to differ from each other. The difference is a function of the context of an utterance. For example, it could be due to the number of segments in an utterance and the feature bundle composition of the segments. Despite these differences, the two levels are related. This relationship is accomplished by the operation of a set of context-sensitive phonological rules which transform one into the other. Mainly, phonological rules serve to relate the underlying forms at the classificatory level to the phonetic output at the phonetic level.

In essence, phonological rules specify the relation between phonetic and phonological representations in the context of a syntactic structure. The phonological rules map the phonetic forms from the underlying phonological forms. Chomsky and Halle suggest (1968, p. 24):

> The hearer makes use of certain cues and certain expectations to determine the syntactic structure and semantic content of an utterance.

> Given a hypothesis as to its syntactic structure—in particular its surface structure—he uses the phonological principles that he controls to determine a phonetic shape. The hypothesis will then be accepted if it is not too radically at variance with the acoustic material, where the range of permitted discrepancy may vary widely with conditions and many individual factors. Given acceptance of such a hypothesis, what the hearer "hears" is what is internally generated by the rules. That is, he will "hear" the phonetic shape determined by the postulated syntactic structure and the internalized rules.

They question the need for the representation to be correct in full detail for a theory of grammar. Recognition of the many performance variables operating on the underlying representation during utterances does not require them to abandon the idea of universal features, only to explain why they vary in speech contexts.

All of these variables, they suggest, are not yet very well understood and perhaps may never need to be understood in order to develop a general linguistic theory. Possibly, the properties of speech which are present, but not essential to the description of the characteristics or properties of any human language, will not get in the way of understanding the essential properties which characterize any human language.

Obviously, linguists' interest in describing the structure of language, rather than the acoustics and physiology of speech, dictate their views of the parameters which are important. For example, Chomsky and Halle do not view phonetic transcription as a device for recording observable attributes in actual language utterances. Instead, they view it as a representation of what the listener concludes the phonetic properties are. In this sense, the phonetic transcription represents the hearer's interpretation, rather than observable properties, of the signal. In short, it is phonemic (broad transcription), instead of phonetic (narrow transcription). They explain (1968, p. 294):

> Thus it is no longer a problem that the transcription is composed of discrete symbols whereas the signal is quasi-continuous, or that the transcription provides information only about some properties of the signal and not about others, or finally, that physically identical signals may have distinct phonetic transcriptions. Clearly, a person's interpretation of a particular speech event is not determined merely by the physical properties constituting the event. A person will normally not be aware of many properties manifest in the signal, and, at the same time, his interpretation may involve elements which have no direct physical correlates, since what is perceived depends not only on the physical constitution of the signal but also on the hearer's knowledge of the language as well as on a host of extra-grammatical factors.

The system they have proposed in their book is basically a competence, not a performance, model. Consequently, Chomsky and Halle describe underlying features and the rules relating them to the actual form in utterances. This is because their efforts are directed toward phonological theory. Nevertheless, they recognize the importance of a performance model for a full description of language. In that recognition, they acknowledge the need to explore some of the variables considered important by other investigators. The competence model, they reflect, generates the rules (and thus, the idealized representations), whereas the performance model includes the grammar (the rules), but also the many other factors that determine the actual physical signal. They suggest (1968, p. 111):

> It must, incidentally, be borne in mind that the specific competence-performance delimitation provided by a grammar represents a hypothesis that might prove to be in error when other factors that play a role in performance and the interrelation of these various factors come under investigation. . . . When a theory of performance ultimately emerges, we may find that some of the facts we are attempting to explain do not really belong to grammar but instead fall under the theory of performance, and that certain facts that we neglect, believing them to be fea-

> tures of performance, should really have been incorporated in the system of grammatical rules.

Thus, Chomsky and Halle join others in recognizing the need for additional research if the nature of distinctive features is to be fully understood. The model they proposed has not been extensively tested, nor has it been unconditionally accepted. Chomsky and Halle admit that the properties they have identified may be modified, changed, or replaced as other variables are explored.

The set of distinctive features proposed by Chomsky and Halle contains some of the features proposed by Jakobson, Fant, and Halle. This overlap of features in proposed distinctive feature systems is not uncommon, whether they are linguistically generated or developed from experimental acoustic and physiological work in speech sound attributes. The overlap is evidence that investigators concur on some of the features which are basic to the English language. In addition, it is an indication that distinctive features, as the basic articulatory elements in phonemes, are becoming more widely accepted.

Because of the similar features composing several distinctive feature systems, any one may be used for analyzing articulation errors. The system used in this text is the one proposed by Chomsky and Halle. Their system has been applied experimentally to children's misarticulations (McReynolds and Huston, 1971; McReynolds and Bennett, 1972). Thus, data on the applicability of Chomsky and Halle's proposed distinctive features for evaluating children's articulation errors are available. Empirical evidence has shown that the system can be used for this purpose.

The next chapter describes the 13 distinctive features of English as proposed by Chomsky and Halle. It is not a comprehensive explanation, and the reader is referred to *The Sound Pattern of English* (Chomsky and Halle, 1968) for more detailed descriptions.

For a detailed description and comparison of the other distinctive feature systems, the reader may refer to *Distinctive Features: Theory and Validation* (Singh, 1975).

3

Distinctive Features Proposed by Chomsky and Halle

Chomsky and Halle propose a universal set of features which represents man's total phonetic capabilities across all languages. For English, some of the features included in the universal set are not relevant. Only 13 features from the universal set are used to describe the phonemes of English. On the classificatory level, these 13 features are binary; each feature is present (marked by a "+") or absent (marked by a "–") in a phoneme. For example, the feature of continuancy is present in the phoneme /ʃ/ but absent in the phoneme /tʃ/. All other features comprising the two phonemes are the same. Since the feature provides the contrast for forming a minimal pair, it functions to differentiate the two phonemes in the English language. In the same manner, the features composing /f/ and /v/ are identical except for one feature, voicing. Voicing is present in /v/ but absent in /f/. Therefore, /f/ is described as "nonvoiced" or (–) voice, and /v/ is described as "voiced" or (+) voice. The phonemes /f/ and /v/ represent a minimal pair. As noted by Chomsky and Halle, "each feature is a physical scale defined by two points, which are designated by antonymous adjectives: high - nonhigh, voiced - nonvoiced. . ." (p. 299).

The 13 distinctive features of English are:

1. Vocalic	Nonvocalic
2. Consonantal	Nonconsonantal
3. Coronal	Noncoronal
4. Anterior	Nonanterior
5. High	Nonhigh
6. Back	Nonback
7. Low	Nonlow
8. Nasal	Nonnasal
9. Round	Nonround
10. Continuant	Noncontinuant
11. Tense	Nontense
12. Voice	Nonvoice
13. Strident	Nonstrident

These 13 features are defined by Chomsky and Halle in terms of articulatory and acoustical properties. The properties are the distinctive features. Chomsky and Halle's complete definitions for each feature are provided in Chapter 7. Some of the features are similar to a "place - manner" description of phonemes.

The first two features–vocalic and consonantal–are referred to as "major class features" since they define the categories of speech sounds. Most phonemes of English are either (+) vocalic and (−) consonantal, or (−) vocalic and (+) consonantal. Only the phonemes /r/ and /l/ are both (+) vocalic and (+) consonantal, whereas the /h/, /w/, and /j/ are both (−) vocalic and (−) consonantal. Both vocalic and consonantal features are defined by the varying aspects of the opening and closing of the vocal tract in speech.

The next seven features—coronal, anterior, high, low, back, nasal, and round—are "cavity features," according to Chomsky and Halle. Some of the features in this group are defined somewhat analogously by the common term "place." For example, the features "high," "low," and "back" refer to the placement of the body of the tongue. The phoneme /p/ is (−) high, (−) back, and (−) low, compared to /k/ which is (+) high, (+) back, and (−) low.

The next two features—continuancy and tenseness—are associated with "manner of articulation." In continuant sounds, ". . . the primary constriction in the vocal tract is not narrowed to the point where the air flow past the constriction is blocked. . ." (p. 317). In noncontinuants, the air flow through the mouth is essentially blocked. Phonemes such as /f/ and /θ/ are continuant phonemes, whereas /p/ and /t/ are noncontinuant phonemes. Tenseness refers to the action of supraglottal musculature during production. Tense phonemes are produced with deliberate and intense musculature effort. Nontense sounds are produced rapidly and in somewhat of a superficial or indistinct manner.

The last two features characterizing English are "voicing" and "stridency," which Chomsky and Halle refer to as "source features." Of all features, the term "voicing" is the most familiar. Vocal cord vibration is present in voicing. Nonvoicing refers to a glottal opening so wide that vocal vibration from air flow through the opening is prevented.

The feature of stridency is characterized by turbulence of air flow as it passes over a surface. "A rougher surface, a faster rate of flow, and an angle of incidence closer to ninety degrees will all contribute to greater stridency" (p. 329). Phonemes such as /s/, /z/, /ʃ/, and /tʃ/ are (+) strident phonemes. Examples of nonstridents are plosives such as /p/ and /b/.

Analyzing a phoneme in terms of features entails listing each feature, since a phoneme is composed of a bundle of features. For example, the feature bundle composing /tʃ/ is:

(−) vocalic
(+) consonantal
(+) high
(−) back
(−) low
(−) anterior
(+) coronal
(−) voice
(−) continuant
(−) nasal
(+) strident

A comparison between two phonemes requires a comparison of each feature composing both of them. In addition to distinguishing two phonemes from each other, features function to separate classes of phonemes. To illustrate, all voiced stops are composed of the following set of features:

(+) consonantal
(−) vocalic
(−) continuant
(−) strident
(+) voice

In effect, the set describes a class of phonemes characterized as voiced stops. The addition of other features to previously formed sets results in the formation of phoneme classes which contrast with other classes. The above set of features, for instance, may separate a class of voiced stops from a class of voiced fricatives or a class of nonvoiced stops.

Further differentiation of the stops within a class requires the addition of other features to form the minimal contrasts between voiced stop consonants. For example, addition of the (+) and (−) coronal contrast separates the /b/ from the /d/ in the set of voiced stops. Generally, when a new feature is added to an individual's repertoire, emergence of several new phonemes is possible. Acquisition of stridency suggests a separation of all (+) strident phonemes from (−) strident phonemes. In principle, the /s/, /z/, /ʃ/, /f/, /v/, /tʃ/, /ʒ/, and /dʒ/ could emerge as a class of (+) strident phonemes distinguished from a class of (−) strident phonemes. Possibly, eight phonemes could be added when (+) stridency is acquired, provided the appropriate basic feature sets have been acquired previously.

4

Application of Distinctive Features to Articulation Errors

Jakobson (1971) suggests that, in learning the phonology of his language, a child does not acquire phonemes as such. His phoneme acquisition is a function of feature contrast acquisition. Jakobson suggests a developmental sequence in feature learning. Furthermore, he assumes that some features, or feature sets, are prerequisites to acquisition of other features and sets. When a child acquires a feature, he has already acquired others which, when formed into sets, make possible the formation of new phonemes. He learns these phonemes because he successively learns to contrast the smallest, distinctive, meaningful units of sounds. These units are the distinctive features.

Because phonemes are composed of bundles of features, minimal feature contrasts are learned progressively. All feature contrasts cannot be learned simultaneously, since the child must be exposed to minimal pairs before he can learn any one feature. As he learns the features successively, more phonemes are added to his articulatory repertoire. Progressively, as a child adds a new feature to his phonological repertoire, he distinguishes between more phoneme classes as well as more phoneme pairs.

Initially, a child distinguishes only a few feature contrasts. The first distinction he makes is the vocalic/consonantal contrast. He acquires vowels and consonants as classes. After he has made this separation, he acquires the nasal/oral (non-nasal) distinction. In this operation he separates the consonant class into two classes on the basis of the nasal/oral feature contrast. Later, he separates both the nasal and oral classes on the basis of place features. In particular, he distinguishes labial consonants from dental consonants in the nasal class of phonemes. In a similar fashion, he distinguishes labial from dental consonants in the oral class. As he acquires more features (and simultaneously, more feature contrasts), he distinguishes new classes of consonants. Finally, distinctions are made between phonemes within a class on the basis of single features. Distinctions may also be made on the basis of more than one feature difference, between classes or single phoneme pairs. For example, acquisition of the nasal/oral and labial/dental separation allows him to learn that /p/ is oral-labial and that /n/ is nasal-dental.

No well executed studies have been conducted to test Jakobson's theory of how children acquire phonology. Some longitudinal observational studies of single children, however, have provided information about their feature acquisition in an indirect fashion (Ferguson and Slobin, 1973; Bar-Adon and Leopold, 1971). Evidence has been supportive of his theory of feature acquisition.

Another source of support for Jakobson's theory is provided by Crocker (1969), who investigated the possibility of constructing a theoretical linguistic model of children's acquisition of phonology. He applied Chomsky and Halle's competence model of English phonology and Jakobson, Fant, and Halle's distinctive features to normative data from several studies of phoneme development. He concluded that children do apply phonological rules in acquiring, combining, and separating distinctive features progressively as they learn the phonemes of their language.

Information concerning children's acquisition of features is limited. However, some evidence has been presented which provides insight into how children learn English phonemes. In turn, this information can be applied to articulation problems. Thus, in addition to studying phonological acquisition, Crocker attempted to determine whether phonological rules would provide a rationale for explaining the sound substitutions of children with articulation errors. His investigation led him to believe that errors are systematic and occur primarily because children fail to apply a particular rule during the developmental sequence.

Investigators suggest that distinctive feature theory may be used to evaluate and explain some children's articulation problems. Several researchers have applied linguistic methods in analyzing and describing children's articulation patterns and deviant phonological systems (Albright and Albright, 1958; Applegate, 1961; Compton, 1970; Haas, 1963). Winitz describes application of distinctive feature theory to articulation in his book *Articulatory Acquisition and Behavior* (1969). Although most of the discussion is devoted to features in phoneme acquisition, he also explores the implications for articulation errors.

A study by Menyuk (1968) contributed further evidence that articulation errors can be described on the basis of distinctive features. She analyzed the distinctive feature content of consonant substitutions made by American and Japanese children during the developmental period, and those made by American children with articulation problems. These were compared to adult consonant substitutions. Features used in the analysis were from those proposed by Jakobson, Fant, and Halle. They included gravity, diffuseness, stridency, nasality, continuancy, and voicing.

Developmentally, she found that both groups of normal children were using consonants which contained the features of (+) nasal, (+) grave, and (+) voice correctly more often than consonants containing the features of (+) diffuse, (+) continuant, and (+) strident. Her results suggest that some features are acquired earlier than others by normally developing children and that probably, as Jakobson proposed, they develop in an orderly sequence. Since both language groups showed similar patterns of acquisition, the findings support the universal nature of distinctive features.

Generally, the children with articulation errors maintained all the features significantly less in their substitutions than did the normally developing children. What is more, it appeared that some of the later appearing features were less well maintained by children with articulation problems than were earlier appearing features. For example, in their error sounds, the children most frequently substituted nonstrident sounds for strident sounds.

The normally developing children maintained voicing most frequently in their substitutions. In descending order they maintained stridency, continuancy, gravity, and diffuseness in their substitutions. On the other hand, children with articulation errors maintained nasality most often. Voicing, gravity, continuancy, diffuseness, and stridency were maintained in that order. Analysis of the feature errors allowed Menyuk to derive the rule by which certain phoneme substitutions would be generated. In turn, it enabled her to predict substitutions that would be produced by a child in the context of various morphemes.

In summary, Menyuk's study indicates the usefulness of describing articulation errors on the basis of feature errors. Her findings stimulate other questions: if a feature is in error in one phoneme, might not other phonemes containing that feature also be in error? To extend this conjecture even further, if a feature is changed in one of the phonemes, will it be changed in the other phonemes as well?

Although in the studies discussed thus far articulation errors were subject to a phonological or distinctive feature analysis, they did not provide a detailed and systematic analysis of all articulation errors; that is, a child's complete articulation profile was not presented. In addition, studies have not evaluated the usefulness of any one distinctive feature system for this purpose.

A more comprehensive exploration in application of one distinctive feature system was completed by McReynolds and Huston (1971). In this study, an analysis procedure using Chomsky and Halle's set of distinctive features, was applied to evaluation of the articulation of children with severe articulation errors. The purpose of the analysis was to investigate whether errors could be described on the basis of consistent feature errors and whether particular features were in error in the children's articulation.

Ten children with severe articulation problems were administered the McDonald Deep Test of Articulation. Their responses to the test items were transcribed and analyzed according to the features proposed by Chomsky and Halle. The features composing the test (target) phonemes and the features composing the responses the child produced were compared. Features maintained in each response and features changed in each response provided data for the feature error analysis.

Results of the study showed that children's articulation errors could be described as *errors in distinctive features.* The feature errors made by the children were consistent across most phonemes which contained that feature. Within the group of 10 children, two types of errors emerged.

For one group, some features were absent entirely in the children's phonological repertoires. They did not produce any phonemes in which these features were present. For example, (+) stridency was completely missing in one child's productions. Seven phonemes were affected: /s/, /z/, /f/, /v/, /tʃ/, /dʒ/, and /ʒ/. For another child, (−) voicing was never produced. Thus, /p/, /t/, /k/, /f/, /θ/, /s/, /ʃ/, and /tʃ/ were in error. Lack of a feature was reflected in eight phoneme errors. Children in the first group did not have all the feature contrasts basic to acquisition of English phonemes. When a feature was lacking, the lack was reflected in a whole class of phonemes.

The other group of children produced all the features. That is, all feature contrasts were produced in their responses, although sometimes in inappropriate sets. Their errors consisted of producing the features in inappropriate contexts or bundles. Essentially, although the feature contrasts were present in these children's repertoires, they were misused.

The descriptive study demonstrated the feasibility of evaluating misarticulations at the level of distinctive features, instead of phonemes. Several aspects of the study deserve mention. First, Chomsky and Halle's distinctive feature system was used successfully in describing articulation errors as errors in features, the articulatory elements underlying phonemes. Second, errors produced by the children were not random. A consistent error pattern across phonemes in which features were present was discovered.

The second finding was interesting in that a provocative aspect of distinctive feature theory is the generalized nature of features. This refers to the fact that a feature is not limited to the composition of one phoneme only; rather, each of the features is present in several phonemes, as for example, (+) voicing. It is present in the consonants /b/, /d/, /g/, /z/, /v/, /ð/, /dʒ/, and /ʒ/. (It is also present in /m/, /n/, and /ŋ/, but does not function in a contrastive manner for them.)

As already noted, according to Jakobson's model, acquisition of a feature provides a child with an opportunity to set up a class of phonemes, not just one phoneme. Thus, *feature acquisition,* as opposed to phoneme acquisition, presents a more economical view of the way children learn the phonemes of their language. Instead of learning one phoneme at a time, or learning each feature individually and separately in each bundle (phoneme), features are acquired across phonemes and feature sets already present. When phonemes are viewed as being acquired individually, the articulatory properties composing one phoneme have little relationship with articulatory properties composing other phonemes. In contrast, feature acquisition suggests a functional relationship between the properties composing various phonemes. More precisely, features acquired in one phoneme contribute and aid in the acquisition of additional phonemes.

In a somewhat reverse manner, results of the descriptive study may be interpreted as supportive of Jakobson's theory that children acquire a class of phonemes when a new feature is added to their repertoire; *i.e.*, several new phonemes are acquired. Findings showed that a feature error affected several phonemes in which that feature was present. In effect, most of the phonemes within a class were in error when a feature was lacking in a child's repertoire. The generalized nature of the feature errors is important for articulation training. Perhaps, if training is directed toward acquisition of a feature, once it has been acquired, the feature may transfer to several of the phonemes in which it is present and in error. More than one phoneme could be changed when a feature is acquired in training. If, indeed, one feature results in changes in several phonemes, the efficiency of articulation training might be enhanced.

Another study was designed to explore whether implications from the descriptive study could be substantiated in an empirical manner (McReynolds and Bennett, 1972). Procedures were developed to obtain information about feature generalization during acquisition. On the basis of feature errors, children from the descriptive study were chosen for the generalization study. Children with different features in error were selected so that the generalization pattern of more than one feature could be explored. The question asked whether training a child to acquire and use a feature in one phoneme would result in transfer of the feature to other untrained phonemes in which it had been in error. In essence, an attempt was made to demonstrate that a distinctive feature is acquired in several phonemes simultaneously.

Programs were designed to train the children to acquire a feature that had been found to be in error on their articulation test. The training programs will not be described in this part since they will be fully detailed in Part III, Developing Training Programs.

During training, frequent assessments were made on selected phonemes and contexts to test generalization of the trained feature to contexts other than the trained one. For example, one of the children received training on (+) stridency. On the phonemes /f/, /v/, /s/, /z/, and /tʃ/ on the McDonald Test he had lacked (+) stridency entirely. These phonemes belong to a class of (+) strident phonemes in that (+) stridency is one of the features present in all of them. From these error phonemes, the /f/ was chosen as the phoneme in which stridency would be trained. When the child had acquired the /f/, generalization was tested by readministering the /f/, /v/, /s/, /z/, and /tʃ/ items from the McDonald Test. Testing the /f/ items enabled exploration of transfer from the nonsense syllables used in training to two-syllable words with /f/ in the releasing and arresting positions. In addition, transfer to the remaining error phonemes was tested, also in the context of words in which the phonemes formed both the releasing and arresting positions.

In general, results of the training study showed that transfer of features occurs. After training on one phoneme, the children transferred the feature to other phonemes. Findings supported the contention that children may acquire several phonemes in the process of acquiring a feature. Not only did the results support phonological theory, they had implications for the way in which some articulation errors should be considered, or viewed, in evaluation and training. These observations and implications will be discussed in the next chapter. Before doing so, however, qualifications need to be made regarding feature generalization in light of the generalization patterns obtained in the study.

Although transfer was obtained, feature generalization was not uniform across all phonemes. For example, one child was trained on (+) continuancy in /ʃ/. After he had acquired the /ʃ/, other (+) continuant phonemes that had been in error were tested to determine if he had transferred (+) continuancy to them. He was administered the 46 items on the McDonald Test for /s/, /z/, /f/, and /v/ phonemes. Results showed that percentage of error on (+) continuancy was reduced on all of the phonemes tested. However, the reduction ranged from 92 per cent to 36 per cent on individual phonemes. That is, he transferred (+) continuancy to 92 per cent of the /s/ items, but only to 36 per cent of the /z/ items. In effect, (+) continuancy transferred more to some feature bundles (some phonemes) than to others.

Another generalization pattern revealed that position of the phoneme in the test item may have been a variable. Each phoneme was tested in the releasing and arresting positions on the McDonald. The children sometimes transferred the trained feature more frequently to items tested in one of the positions than to items tested in the other position.

It appeared that transfer of a specific feature may be influenced by the features composing the test phoneme as well as the phonetic environment of the test phoneme. That is to say, one or more of the features composing a test phoneme may have an effect on the degree to which a particular feature will generalize. Furthermore, the surrounding phonemes (feature bundles) may also influence generalization of a feature. Obtaining different generalization patterns suggested that additional research needs to be conducted to explore how features influence one another.

5

Distinctive Feature Procedures and Other Articulation Procedures

Returning to consideration of using a distinctive feature analysis for assessing articulation errors requires some discussion of how it differs from other assessment methods. In this chapter, distinctive feature analysis is discussed in relation to the more conventional and popular methods used in evaluating articulation errors and developing treatment programs.

ARTICULATION SAMPLE

Obtaining an articulation sample is basic to all evaluation procedures. The sample may be obtained in a variety of contexts. Sometimes speech pathologists listen to children's spontaneous speech to determine sounds in error. The most frequently used procedure usually entails administration of one of the many articulation tests available on the market. As a basis for a distinctive feature analysis, too, the speech pathologist may use a test, or obtain a spontaneous speech sample. Thus, a distinctive feature approach need not differ from other approaches in the manner in which a child's articulation is sampled.

Conventionally, the articulation tests are constructed so that each phoneme is tested three times, once in initial, once in final, and once in the medial position in a word. Some tests provide an opportunity to elicit imitations of phonemes in isolation and in more complex contexts. Others are designed to obtain spontaneous productions in semi-structured situations by having a child describe pictures. The more comprehensive tests may sample a phoneme more than three times, as for example, when blends are included in the test. Generally, standard tests seldom obtain more than five responses on each of the phonemes tested. In testing for phoneme errors, this sample size is evidently considered sufficient for a reliable estimate of the stability of a child's phoneme errors.

Some exceptions to a limited sample have been proposed in recent years. For instance, McDonald (1964) has suggested that a child's articulation should be tested in a variety of contexts. Shelton and his colleagues have developed the Sound Production Tasks within a similar framework (Elbert, Shelton, and Arndt, 1967; Shelton, Elbert, and Arndt, 1967). In their test, imitation of each phoneme is tested in 30 items in a variety of contexts ranging from isolated sounds to sounds in phrases. Likewise, individuals developing programmed instruction for specific phoneme training suggest a more extensive baseline on the phoneme in error (McLean, 1970). Evidently, individuals are becoming more aware of the need to obtain a large and varied sample as evidence that an error is consistent in a child's articulation (Turton, 1973).

Perhaps a limited sample would be sufficient for a distinctive feature analysis. Since it involves description of a child's entire phonological system, however, a larger sample is desirable, if not mandatory. Features are basic articulatory elements, and each is present in several phonemes. Not only may a child produce a feature in the context of one phoneme and not another, but, as the generalization data showed, he may sometimes produce it in a phoneme in one context while omitting it in the same phoneme in another context (McReynolds and Bennett, 1972). In order to place confidence in statements concerning the presence or absence of the basic elements in a child's articulation, the sample should be large enough to evidence stability of the feature. If lawfulness in feature use is being explored, a 3-response sample is probably too restricted. In the research reported in this text, 46 responses to each consonant formed the sample. It provided from 200 to more than 400 samples of each feature; this very large sample allowed conclusions to be drawn about feature production by each child. For clinical purposes, this sample size may be larger than is needed. Since the original study, a number of children with six or more phonemes in error have served as subjects in other distinctive feature studies. An examination of their McDonald profiles shows that a stable response pattern may be obtained frequently in the first 10 items of the test. Therefore, for children with severe articulation errors, a sample of 10 responses to each phoneme would probably be sufficient to allow a reliable distinctive feature analysis to be conducted.

In summary, the means for sampling articulation for a distinctive feature analysis need not be different from the means used for conventional approaches. However, the speech pathologist is encouraged to enlarge the size of the sample for each phoneme when contemplating a distinctive feature analysis. As already noted, it is recommended that each phoneme be tested approximately 10 times. Extension of the sample to a larger size is somewhat dependent on the degree of specificity with which the speech pathologist desires the child's phonological system to be described. In principle, the more specific and detailed the description, the larger the size of the sample, and the greater the contextual variety from which it is obtained.

METHOD FOR RECORDING ARTICULATION RESPONSES

The methods for recording children's articulation responses may take one of several forms. They range from simple notations to detailed and complex ones. At the least complex level, the speech pathologist may choose to score responses as simply correct or incorrect rather than specify what constitutes an incorrect response. At another level, the speech pathologist might record incorrect responses as distortions, substitutions, or omissions. This system provides more information about the form of incorrect responses in that they are placed into one of three possible categories. However, the specific distortion and substitution may not be described within these categories. Finally, recording may involve transcription of the child's articulation as he responds to the test phoneme. At this level the child's production is specified. The speech pathologist may use either phonemic (broad) transcription or phonetic (narrow) transcription in recording.

The method used may depend on the

speech pathologist's approach to training. It may also be related to the criteria for selecting the sound to be trained. These two aspects are discussed in the next two sections of the chapter.

Only one of the recording methods is possible if a distinctive feature analysis is to be conducted. A distinctive feature analysis requires specification or identification of the child's production. For this reason, the child's responses to the test phoneme must be transcribed.

If the features used in the analysis are those proposed as linguistically relevant features, the clinician will most likely use phonemic or broad transcription. Other features present in the productions may not be recorded. On the other hand, if the analysis uses features which can be identified even though they are not linguistically relevant, the clinician may choose to use phonetic or narrow transcription. Regardless of the system used, a feature analysis requires that the clinician be able to specify which features the child is producing. This can be accomplished only if the sounds produced by the child are identified. The clinician must examine the sounds produced by the child to determine which features are being produced.

In summary, several methods of recording responses are possible with some approaches to articulation evaluation and treatment. A distinctive feature analysis, however, requires that the speech pathologist transcribe the child's responses during the sampling procedure. This is necessary because it is essential that the features produced by the child be identified.

SELECTION OF A PHONEME FOR TRAINING

Probably the most frequently used criterion for phoneme selection is information from developmental data (Poole, 1934; Templin, 1957; Wellman, Case, Mengert, and Bradbury, 1931). Age is taken into consideration, and phonemes are selected for training on the basis of appearance at specific ages. Sometimes speech pathologists consider consistency of the error (Sprietersbach and Curtis, 1951; McDonald, 1964), or frequency of occurrence of the error phoneme in the language (Wood, 1949) when deciding which phoneme should be trained. Stimulability is often added to the list of criteria to be taken into consideration (Snow and Milisen, 1954; Farquhar, 1961). If a child can imitate some of the target sounds, but not others, he may receive training first on those he can imitate. At times, practical considerations enter into selection criteria. If group training is scheduled, children with several phonemes in error may be administered training on a phoneme that other children also misarticulate.

Probably most speech pathologists take several of these criteria into consideration in selecting training phonemes. Thus, selection of target phonemes may be based on one or several parameters, some of which are dependent on the speech pathologist's approach to articulation problems.

The above criteria are related to the child's articulation to different degrees of directness. That is, some are related more closely to what the child is doing during testing than are others. For example, when stimulability is used as a criterion, the clinician assesses the child's ability to imitate. In this, he uses an attribute inherent in the child's response for selecting a target phoneme. Developmental data, on the other hand, are related less directly to what the child is actually producing during evaluation. In this case, the child's age is the primary consideration. Selecting to train a particular phoneme because children are needed to fill a group is related only remotely to the child's total articulation performance. Basically, these criteria are derived only partly from the properties of the child's articulation during assessment. Consequently, they involve principles different from the principle involved in selecting a phoneme on the basis of a distinctive feature analysis.

Somewhat in contrast to the above mentioned criteria, a distinctive feature analysis requires consideration of the parameters constituting each of the child's productions. What is more, the presence of each feature across all phonemes is examined, and a target sound is selected on the basis of features the child is and is not producing. To accomplish this, features composing his productions are compared to the features composing each test phoneme in each context in the articulation sample. In short, features of the child's productions are compared to features of the target phonemes. This procedure is necessary to obtain information for selecting a training phoneme in that the comparison shows which features match and which features mismatch in the two. Identification of the correctly and incorrectly produced features allows the correctly produced ones to be used as a foundation for training the features in error. In this manner, they function as facilitating environments for training features. To state it another way, comparison enables specification of the phonological rules operating in the child's articulation. Training phonemes are selected in the expectation that they will function to change the rules. Essentially, then, the selected phoneme is composed of features the child already has in his repertoire, plus the feature he is to acquire. Both of these can be specified only if the content of the child's productions are described in detail. That is, phoneme selection is based almost entirely on the articulatory properties present and absent in the child's phoneme productions.

To illustrate the principle described above, a somewhat broad example is presented. The phonemes /s/, /z/, /ʃ/, /f/, /v/, and /ʒ/ are (+) continuant and (+) strident. Other features also compose them, and (+) stridency and (+) continuancy are just two of the features. Each of the phonemes, however, is composed of somewhat different features. During testing, the child may substitute other phonemes for some of them. He may, for example, produce /tʃ/ for /s/, /ʃ/, /f/, and /v/, and substitute /d/ for /z/. Since /tʃ/ is (+) strident but (−) continuant, and /d/ is also (−) continuant, it appears that a phonological rule operating rather consistently in the child's production is that (+) strident and (+) continuant phonemes are changed to (+) strident and (−) continuant phonemes. The rule is expressed thusly:

$$\begin{bmatrix} (+)\text{ continuant} \\ (+)\text{ strident} \end{bmatrix} \longrightarrow \begin{bmatrix} (-)\text{ continuant} \\ (+)\text{ strident} \end{bmatrix}$$

This change may occur across most of the (+) strident and (+) continuant phonemes tested. After a complete analysis, it may become clear that the child needs training on a phoneme which will provide him with the feature (+) continuancy, so that he may make a separation between the class of (+) strident, (+) continuant phonemes and a class of (+) strident, (−) continuant phonemes. The speech pathologist would therefore select a (+) strident and (+) continuant phoneme for training.

As shown in the example, a training phoneme is selected on the basis of the child's productions of the test sounds in comparison to the standard sounds. Although the example is somewhat general, it demonstrates the difference between a distinctive feature analysis and other approaches for selection of a phoneme for training. A complete analysis would consider other variables in addition to those described. These will be discussed in Chapters 13 and 14 in Part III.

TRAINING PRINCIPLES

In articulation treatment, training is directed toward teaching children to articulate their error phonemes correctly. If a child has several phonemes in error, the clinician selects one to train initially. When the child has acquired that phoneme, the speech pathologist selects a second phoneme to train. Selection of new target phonemes continues until each of the child's error phonemes has been corrected.

Phonemes are trained in a distinctive feature approach also. Theoretically, however, the emphasis is placed on acquisition of a feature contrast rather than just the phoneme on which training is administered. Recall, when features are in error, it customarily means that a child produces only phonemes having the (+) aspect, or only phonemes having the (−) aspect of the feature. Training, then, is directed toward acquisition of both the (+) and (−) aspects of the feature. Of course, the contrast cannot be trained independently. That is, a feature contrast can only be trained in the context of phonemes in which each aspect is present. Specifically, training should involve two phonemes, one in which the (+) aspect of the feature is present and one in which the (−) aspect is present.

Ideally, the two phonemes are selected because they form a minimal pair. In other words, they consist of identical features except for the feature requiring training. An example would be /p/ and /b/ for training a child in the voicing contrast. The /p/ and /b/ share the same features except for voicing. The /p/ is (−) voiced and the /b/ is (+) voiced. By presenting a minimal pair in training, it is hoped that the feature contrast is enhanced. The contrast might then be acquired more readily than if the contrast is presented in the context of phonemes which differ from each other by several features. In theory, minimal contrast training parallels the suggested manner in which normal phonological acquisition takes place and therefore appears logical in training.

Since training is directed toward teaching a child to acquire a feature contrast rather than the training phoneme alone, a distinctive feature analysis places emphasis on the importance of relationships among phonemes. That is, a distinctive feature approach is not conducive to viewing each phoneme error as an independent one. Instead, the fact that a feature is present in several phonemes suggests that transfer of the feature should occur across phonemes as the child acquires the contrast. Therefore, in distinctive feature training, the speech pathologist is alerted to explore whether changes are occurring on other phonemes in which the feature is present. That is to say, generalization across phonemes is an expected occurrence, and other phonemes are under constant surveillance. Periodically, during the training program, the child's articulation of phonemes not receiving training is tested. If anticipated generalization occurs and the speech pathologist is alert to it, training may take less time. In other words, some of the untrained error sounds may change without training when a feature contrast is trained in the context of one phoneme pair.

In summary, although phonemes are trained as in other conventional articulation programs, emphasis in distinctive feature training is placed on training a feature contrast in the context of two phonemes. Theoretically, acquisition of a feature should result in generalization of the feature across some of the phonemes in which the feature is present and in error.

6

Summary to Part I

This part was a general introduction to the role of distinctive feature theory in the treatment of articulation disorders. A brief theoretical background was included to demonstrate the relevance of distinctive features to articulation and to articulation errors. The relationship between the two was examined partly by describing differences between a distinctive feature approach and other approaches to articulation evaluation and training.

For individuals with no background in linguistics, Part I may have seemed difficult. If this part was not clear, it is suggested that individuals proceed to the second part. Completing the exercises in the remainder of the book may be more helpful than a second reading of Part I at this stage. Working through an analysis of a child's misarticulations can be enlightening. It sometimes functions to define the features more concisely, thus clearing up confusion about the principles involved in distinctive feature theory. After completing the exercises, a second reading of Part I may prove more fruitful.

II

PROCEDURES FOR A DISTINCTIVE FEATURE ANALYSIS OF ARTICULATION ERRORS

The purpose of this part is to present procedures for completing a distinctive feature analysis of children's articulation errors. The part is divided into six chapters. Chapter 7 presents definitions of the 13 features comprising the distinctive feature system proposed by Chomsky and Halle. Chapter 8 provides instructions for using their table to determine features composing each consonant and vowel in the English language. Requirements of an articulation sample suitable for a distinctive feature analysis are discussed in Chapter 9. Chapters 10 and 11 present specific procedures for completing worksheets and analysis sheets for a distinctive feature analysis. Preparation of a distinctive feature summary sheet is described in Chapter 12.

Articulation test results for two children are included in this part for teaching the analysis procedure. The first child's articulation errors are used for teaching each procedure in the analysis. The second child's articulation errors can be used to complete an analysis without additional direct training on each procedure and for practice on a smaller articulation sample.

The material in this part is arranged in a programmed manner. At the end of each chapter are exercises. The exercises provide training for completing the procedures employed in each level of the analysis. Answers to the exercises are located at the end of each chapter. Completing each exercise correctly, before going on to the next chapter, will facilitate learning the distinctive feature analysis.

7

Chomsky and Halle's Distinctive Feature Definitions

Definitions for the 13 distinctive features proposed by Chomsky and Halle (1968) are presented in Table 1. As previously stated, on a classificatory level, their distinctive feature system is a binary one. All of the distinctive features are either positive (+) or negative (−) in that the feature is either present (+) or absent (−) in a phoneme. The definitions presented in Table 1 are based on the (+) or positive aspect of the feature contrast. All of the phonemes listed after each definition contain the (+) aspect of the feature contrast. For example, when the vocalic feature is present in a phoneme, the articulatory and acoustical characteristics described in the definition are present. In addition, all 15 phonemes listed after the definition contain those articulatory and acoustical characteristics. A phoneme not listed after the definition usually contains the (−) or negative aspect of the feature contrast. However, there are a few features which are irrelevant to some phonemes. In this case, neither the (+) or (−) aspect is present in that phoneme. For example, the features of round and tense are irrelevant features for consonants.

As shown in Table 1, each distinctive feature is present in more than one phoneme. This is indicated by the number of phonemes listed at the end of each definition. In other words, phonemes share many of the same features. It is the particular combination of features and feature aspects that identifies specific phonemes.

Table 1. Definitions of the 13 distinctive features proposed by Chomsky and Halle (*The Sound Pattern of English*, 1968, pages 302–329)

1. *Vocalic.* Two conditions are necessary for a sound to be labeled vocalic: the constriction in the oral cavity cannot be greater than that required for the /i/ and /u/, and the vocal cords must be positioned to allow spontaneous voicing. Vocalic sounds include the liquids and the vowels. They are the /i/, /u/, /eɪ/, /ou/, /aɪ/, /ɔɪ/, /ɪ/, /ʊ/, /ɛ/, /o/, /ɔ/, /r/, /l/, /æ/, and /ʌ/. (Negative: nonvocalic.)

2. *Consonantal.* Consonantal sounds are made with a narrow constriction as in the fricative consonants. All liquids, nasal consonants, and nonnasal consonants have this feature. Consonants include the /r/, /l/, /p/, /b/, /r/, /v/, /ð/, /θ/, /t/, /k/, /g/, /m/, /t/, /d/, /ʃ/, /dʒ/, /n/, /s/, /z/, /ʒ/, and /ŋ/. (Negative: nonconsonantal.)

(continued next page)

3. *Rounded.* A narrowing of the lip orifice is a characterization of a rounded sound. They include the /u/, /ou/, /w/, /ɔɪ/, /ɤ/, /o/, and /ɔ/. (Negative: nonround.)

4. *Tense.* Tense sounds are produced with considerable effort by supraglottal musculature in that the articulatory organs maintain their configurations for a relatively long period. The tense feature is present in the /i/, /u/, /eɪ/, /ou/, /aɪ/, and /ɔɪ/. (Negative: nontense.)

5. *Nasal.* When the velum is lowered to allow the air to be directed through the nose, the nasal feature is present. The sounds with this feature include the /m/, /n/, and /ŋ/. (Negative: nonnasal.)

6. *Continuant.* In a continuant sound a partial obstruction to the air flow is present in the vocal tract. Continuants include the /l/, /r/, /f/, /v/, /θ/, /ð/, /s/, /z/, /ʃ/, /ʒ/, and /h/. (Negative: noncontinuant.)

7. *Voiced.* In voiced sounds the vocal cords are vibrating. The /r/, /l/, /b/, /d/, /v/, /g/, /z/, /m/, /n/, /ð/, /ʒ/, /d /, and /ŋ/ have the feature of voicing. (Negative: nonvoiced.)

8. *Strident.* A strident sound is characterized by noisiness which is produced when air is passed over a rough surface at the necessary rate of flow and angle of incidence. The phonemes /f/, /v/, /s/, /z/, /ʃ/, /tʃ/, /ʒ/, and /dʒ/ are phonemes which have a strident feature. (Negative: nonstrident.)

9. *Coronal.* In coronal sounds the blade of the tongue is raised from the neutral position. The coronal feature is included in the /r/, /l/, /t/, /d/, /θ/, /ð/, /n/, /s/, /z/, /ʃ/, /tʃ/, /ʒ/, and /dʒ/. (Negative: noncoronal.)

10. *High.* In the high feature the body of the tongue is raised above the neutral position. The phonemes in which the high position is positive include the /i/, /u/, /I/, /ɤ/, /w/, /j/, /tʃ/, /dʒ/, /k/, /g/, /ʃ/, /ʒ/, and /ŋ/. (Negative: nonhigh.)

11. *Low.* In the low feature the body of the tongue is lowered below the neutral position. The sounds with this feature include the /aɪ/, /ɔɪ/, /æ/, /ɔ/, and /h/. (Negative: nonlow.)

12. *Back.* When the body of the tongue is retracted from the neutral position, the sound includes a back feature. The sounds are /u/, /ou/, /aɪ/, /ɔɪ/, /ɤ/, /ʌ/, /o/, /ɔ/, /w/, /k/, /g/, and /ŋ/. (Negative: nonback.)

13. *Anterior.* The anterior feature is present when a sound is produced in the front region of the mouth in front of where the /ʃ/ is produced. These sounds are the /l/, /p/, /b/, /f/, /v/, /m/, /t/, /d/, /θ/, /ð/, /n/, /s/, and /z/. (Negative: nonanterior.)

EXERCISES

A. Using Table 1, list the phonemes which are (+) strident.

B. Define the feature of (+) anterior.

ANSWERS TO EXERCISES

A. The following phonemes are (+) strident: /f/, /v/, /s/, /z/, /ʃ/, /tʃ/, /dʒ/, and /ʒ/.

B. The feature (+) anterior is present when the phoneme is produced in the front of the mouth in front of where the /ʃ/ is produced.

8

Chomsky and Halle's Distinctive Feature Chart

The Chomsky and Halle Distinctive Feature Chart presented in Table 2 lists the (+) and (−) aspects for each consonant and vowel of the English language. The manner in which the chart is organized provides ready access to the feature composition of each phoneme. It is particularly useful for completing the worksheet used in the distinctive feature analysis and will be used frequently in the analysis.

The left half of the chart specifies the features composing consonants, and the right half specifies the features of vowels. The (+) or (−) aspect of each feature is specified in the column below each consonant and vowel. For example, the first consonant on the chart is the /r/ phoneme. In the column below the /r/ are the feature aspects which compose the /r/:

	/r/
vocalic	(+)
consonantal	(+)
high	(−)
back	(−)
low	(−)
anterior	(−)
coronal	(+)
voice	(+)
continuant	(+)
nasal	(−)
strident	(−)

For most consonants, round and tense are not relevant features. Likewise, the features of voicing, stridency, continuancy, and nasality are not distinctive for differentiating vowels from each other.

Besides showing the (+) and (−) feature aspects of each phoneme, the chart also allows for a comparison of features between phonemes. For example, the phonemes /f/ and /z/ share nine of the same distinctive features. Both phonemes are (−) vocalic, (+) consonantal, (−) high, (−) back, (−) low, (+) anterior, (+) continuant, (−) nasal, and (+) strident. The two phonemes differ on feature aspects of coronal and voice. The phoneme /f/ is (−) coronal and (−) voice whereas /z/ is (+) coronal and (+) voice.

Table 2. Chomsky-Halle distinctive feature chart.

	r	l	p	b	f	v	m	t	d	θ	ð	n	s	z	tʃ	dʒ	ʃ	ʒ	k	g	ŋ	h	i	u	eɪ	ou	aɪ	ɔɪ	ɪ	ʊ	ɛ	ʌ	o	æ	ɔ	w	j
Vocalic	+	+	–	–	–	–	–	–	–	–	–	–	–	–	–	–	–	–	–	–	–	–	+	+	+	+	+	+	+	+	+	+	+	+	+	–	–
Consonantal	+	+	+	+	+	+	+	+	+	+	+	+	+	+	+	+	+	+	+	+	+	–	–	–	–	–	–	–	–	–	–	–	–	–	–	–	–
High	–	–	–	–	–	–	–	–	–	–	–	–	–	–	+	+	+	+	+	+	+	–	+	+	–	–	–	–	+	+	–	–	–	–	–	+	+
Back	–	–	–	–	–	–	–	–	–	–	–	–	–	–	–	–	–	–	+	+	+	–	–	+	–	+	+	+	–	+	–	+	+	–	+	+	–
Low	–	–	–	–	–	–	–	–	–	–	–	–	–	–	–	–	–	–	–	–	–	+	–	–	–	–	+	+	–	–	–	–	–	+	+	–	–
Anterior	–	+	+	+	+	+	+	+	+	+	+	+	+	+	–	–	–	–	–	–	–	–	–	–	–	–	–	–	–	–	–	–	–	–	–	–	–
Coronal	+	+	–	–	–	–	–	+	+	+	+	+	+	+	+	+	+	+	–	–	–	–	–	–	–	–	–	–	–	–	–	–	–	–	–	–	–
Round																							–	+	–	+	–	+	–	+	–	–	+	–	+	+	–
Tense																							+	+	+	+	+	+	–	–	–	–	–	–	–	–	–
Voice	+	+	–	+	–	+	+	–	+	–	+	+	–	+	–	+	–	+	–	+	+	–															
Continuant	+	+	–	–	+	+	–	–	–	+	+	–	+	+	–	–	+	+	–	–	–	+															
Nasal	–	–	–	–	–	–	+	–	–	–	–	+	–	–	–	–	–	–	–	–	+	–															
Strident	–	–	–	–	+	+	–	–	–	–	–	–	+	+	+	+	+	+	–	–	–	–															

EXERCISES

A. Using Table 2, list the features which compose the phoneme /p/.
B. Write the features composing the /θ/ phoneme.
C. List the features composing /w/.
D. Specify the features that differentiate /tʃ/ from /ʃ/.
E. List the feature aspects /ʃ/ and /s/ have in common.
F. Write the features which /r/ and /w/ share.

ANSWERS TO EXERCISES

A. The features of /p/ are:
(–) vocalic
(+) consonantal
(–) high
(–) back
(–) low
(+) anterior
(–) coronal
(–) voice
(–) continuant
(–) nasal
(–) strident

B. The features of /θ/ are:
(–) vocalic
(+) consonantal
(–) high
(–) back
(–) low
(+) anterior
(+) coronal
(–) voice
(+) continuant
(–) nasal
(–) strident

C. The features of /w/ are:
(–) vocalic
(–) consonantal
(+) high
(+) back
(–) low
(–) anterior
(–) coronal
(+) round
(–) tense

D. /tʃ/ and /ʃ/ are differentiated by the following features:
/tʃ/ is (–) continuant
/ʃ/ is (+) continuant

E. The following features are shared by /ʃ/ and /s/:
(–) vocalic

(+) consonantal
(−) back
(−) low
(+) coronal
(−) voice
(+) continuant
(−) nasal
(+) strident

F. The following features are shared by /r/ and /w/:
(−) low
(−) anterior

9

Articulation Sample

To compute a distinctive feature analysis, a somewhat comprehensive sample of the child's articulation should be obtained. The articulation sample may be obtained from spontaneous speech, or from responses to items on an articulation test. Regardless of the source for the sample, it is important that each phoneme be sampled a number of times. A reliable and representative profile of the child's articulation is necessary.

Many articulation tests sample each phoneme three times, once in the initial, once in the final, and once in the medial position of words. For a distinctive feature analysis, such a limited sample makes it difficult to determine with confidence that a child is making consistent errors on features across all the phonemes in which they are present and in the variety of contexts in which phonemes may occur. In a distinctive feature analysis, the speech pathologist is attempting to look for systematic patterns of feature errors in a child's articulation repertoire. Thus, both appropriate and inappropriate use are noted in the analysis. This in-depth analysis requires that a number of responses for each target phoneme be available. Consequently, it is suggested that each phoneme be sampled more than once in each position.

The articulation samples presented in this chapter consist of children's responses to the items on the McDonald Deep Test of Articulation (1964). This test is used because each phoneme is sampled in approximately 46 contexts: 24 times in the arresting position and 22 times in the releasing position. Nineteen consonants and nine vowels are sampled on the McDonald Deep Test, thereby providing extensive data for a distinctive feature analysis.

It is not always necessary to obtain such a complete sample of articulation in order to complete a reliable distinctive feature analysis. If a child produces a consistent error pattern on a sample of 10 items, it is probably not necessary to continue to present additional test items. On the other hand, if a child's responses to the 10 items evidence variability in the substitutions he produces, the number of test items should be increased. Most children, however, will show a systematic pattern after approximately 10 responses for each test phoneme.

A distinctive feature analysis requires that a child's responses be transcribed. It is not sufficient simply to check whether a production is "correct" or "incorrect." Using the IPA, or a similar symbol system, the child's responses are recorded as a correct phoneme, a substituted phoneme, or an omission. The response is specified exactly so that the features composing the test phoneme and the response produced by the child can be compared. To accomplish a comparison, the child's production should be transcribed. If a production is a distortion whose features cannot be specified, it is necessary to delete the production from the analysis, score it as an omission, or use another feature system in the analysis.

Table 3 presents the articulation responses from a child (Child 1) for all phonemes tested on the McDonald Deep Test. His articulation data will be used to teach the procedures for completing a distinctive feature analysis.

Table 3. Articulation test responses from the McDonald Deep Test of Articulation for Child 1

Test Phoneme /p/			Test Phoneme /t/			Test Phoneme /s/			Test Phoneme /v/		
Arresting position		Releasing position	Arresting position		Releasing position	Arresting position		Releasing position	Arresting position		Releasing position
p	1	b	t	1	t	θ	1	θ	b	1	b
p	2	b	d	2	k	θ	2	ð	b	2	b
b	3	b	d	3	k	θ	3	ð	b	3	b
b	4	b	d	4	k	θ	4	θ	b	4	b
p	5	b	t	5	t	θ	5	ð	b	5	m
p	6	b	d	6	t	θ	6	ð	m	6	b
b	7	p	—	7	k	θ	7	ð	b	7	b
b	8	b	—	8	k	θ	8	θ	b	8	b
b	9	b	d	9	t	θ	9	ð	m	9	b
b	10	b	d	10	k	—	10	ð	b	10	b
b	11	p	d	11	t	—	11	ð	b	11	b
b	12	b	t	12	t	θ	12	ð	b	12	m
p	13	b	d	13	d	θ	13	ð	b	13	b
p	14	b	d	14	k	θ	14	ð	b	14	—
b	15	p	t	15	k	θ	15	ð	b	15	—
b	16	p	—	16	k	—	16	ð	b	16	b
b	17	b	—	17	k	—	17	ð	m	17	b
b	18	b	—	18	k	θ	18	ð	b	18	b
b	19	b	t	19	t	—	19	ð	b	19	b
b	20	b	d	20	t	θ	20	ð	b	20	b
b	21	b	d	21	k	θ	21	ð	b	21	b
b	22	b	d	22	k	θ	22	ð	b	22	b
b	23		d	23		θ	23		b	23	
b	24		d	24		θ	24		b	24	

Test phoneme /b/			Test phoneme /d/			Test phoneme /k/			Test phoneme /g/		
Arresting position		Releasing position	Arresting position		Releasing position	Arresting position		Releasing position	Arresting position		Releasing position
b	1	b	d	1	d	k	1	d	g	1	d
b	2	b	d	2	d	k	2	d	g	2	d
b	3	b	d	3	d	k	3	d	g	3	d

Test phoneme /b/			Test phoneme /d/			Test phoneme /k/			Test phoneme /g/		
Arresting position		Releasing position	Arresting position		Releasing position	Arresting position		Releasing position	Arresting position		Releasing position
b	4	b	d	4	d	k	4	d	g	4	d
b	5	b	d	5	d	k	5	d	g	5	d
b	6	b	d	6	d	k	6	d	g	6	d
b	7	b	d	7	d	k	7	d	g	7	d
b	8	b	d	8	d	k	8	d	g	8	d
b	9	b	d	9	d	k	9	d	g	9	d
b	10	b	d	10	d	k	10	d	g	10	d
b	11	b	d	11	d	k	11	d	g	11	d
b	12	b	d	12	d	k	12	d	g	12	d
b	13	b	d	13	d	k	13	d	g	13	d
b	14	b	d	14	d	k	14	d	g	14	d
b	15	b	d	15	d	k	15	d	g	15	d
b	16	b	d	16	d	k	16	d	g	16	d
b	17	b	d	17	d	k	17	d	g	17	d
b	18	b	d	18	d	k	18	d	g	18	d
b	19	b	d	19	d	k	19	d	g	19	d
b	20	b	d	20	d	k	20	d	g	20	d
b	21	b	d	21	d	k	21	d	g	21	d
b	22	b	d	22	d	k	22	d	g	22	d
b	23		d	23		k	23		g	23	
b	24		d	24		k	24		g	24	

Test phoneme /m/			Test phoneme /n/			Test phoneme /l/			Test phoneme /r/		
Arresting position		Releasing position	Arresting position		Releasing position	Arresting position		Releasing position	Arresting position		Releasing position
m	1	m	n	1	n	–	1	l	–	1	w
m	2	m	n	2	n	–	2	l	–	2	w
m	3	m	n	3	n	–	3	l	–	3	w
m	4	m	n	4	n	–	4	l	–	4	w
m	5	m	n	5	n	–	5	l	–	5	w
m	6	m	n	6	n	–	6	l	–	6	w
m	7	m	n	7	n	–	7	l	–	7	w
m	8	m	n	8	n	–	8	l	–	8	w
m	9	m	n	9	n	–	9	l	–	9	w
m	10	m	n	10	n	–	10	l	–	10	w
m	11	m	n	11	n	–	11	l	–	11	w
m	12	m	n	12	n	l	12	l	–	12	w
m	13	m	n	13	n	–	13	l	–	13	w
m	14	m	n	14	n	–	14	l	–	14	w
m	15	m	n	15	n	l	15	l	–	15	w
m	16	m	n	16	n	–	16	l	–	16	w
m	17	m	n	17	n	–	17	l	–	17	w

Test phoneme /m/			Test phoneme /n/			Test phoneme /l/			Test phoneme /r/		
Arresting position		Releasing position	Arresting position		Releasing position	Arresting position		Releasing position	Arresting position		Releasing position
m	18	m	n	18	n	–	18	l	–	18	w
m	19	m	n	19	n	–	19	l	–	19	w
m	20	m	n	20	n	l	20	l	–	20	w
m	21	m	n	21	n	–	21	l	–	21	w
m	22	m	n	22	n	–	22	l	–	22	w
m	23		n	23		–	23		–	23	
m	24		n	24		–	24		–	24	

Test phoneme /f/			Test phoneme /θ/			Test phoneme /z/			Test phoneme /ʃ/		
Arresting position		Releasing position	Arresting position		Releasing position	Arresting position		Releasing position	Arresting position		Releasing position
v	1	w	t	1	d	d	1	d	d	1	d
v	2	w	t	2	d	–	2	d	d	2	d
v	3	w	d	3	d	–	3	d	g	3	g
v	4	w	t	4	d	d	4	d	d	4	g
v	5	w	d	5	d	d	5	d	t	5	–
v	6	w	d	6	d	d	6	d	t	6	g
v	7	w	d	7	d	–	7	d	g	7	g
v	8	w	t	8	d	d	8	d	g	8	–
v	9	w	t	9	d	d	9	d	g	9	–
v	10	w	d	10	d	d	10	d	g	10	g
v	11	w	t	11	d	d	11	d	t	11	g
v	12	w	d	12	d	–	12	d	d	12	g
v	13	w	t	13	d	–	13	d	d	13	g
v	14	w	t	14	d	d	14	d	d	14	–
v	15	w	d	15	d	d	15	d	d	15	g
v	16	w	d	16	d	–	16	d	d	16	g
v	17	w	d	17	d	d	17	d	d	17	g
v	18	w	t	18	d	d	18	d	d	18	g
v	19	w	d	19	d	–	19	d	d	19	g
v	20	w	d	20	d	–	20	d	d	20	g
v	21	w	d	21	d	d	21	d	d	21	–
v	22	w	d	22	d	d	22	d	d	22	g
v	23		d	23		d	23		d	23	
v	24		d	24		d	24		d	24	

Test phoneme /tʃ/			Test phoneme /dʒ/			Test phoneme /ŋ/			Test phoneme /i/		
Arresting position		Releasing position	Arresting position		Releasing position	Arresting position		Releasing position	Arresting position		Releasing position
—	1	d	v	1	d	ŋ	1		i	1	
—	2	d	v	2	d	ŋ	2		i	2	
—	3	d	v	3	d	ŋ	3		i	3	
—	4	d	v	4	d	ŋ	4		i	4	
—	5	d	v	5	d	ŋ	5		i	5	
—	6	d	v	6	d	ŋ	6		i	6	
—	7	d	v	7	d	ŋ	7		i	7	
—	8	d	v	8	d	ŋ	8		i	8	
d	9	d	v	9	d	ŋ	9		i	9	
d	10	d	v	10	d	ŋ	10		i	10	
d	11	d	v	11	d	ŋ	11		i	11	
—	12	d	v	12	d	ŋ	12		i	12	
—	13	d	v	13	d	ŋ	13		i	13	
—	14	d	v	14	d	ŋ	14		i	14	
d	15	d	v	15	d	ŋ	15		i	15	
d	16	d	v	16	d	ŋ	16		i	16	
—	17	d	v	17	d	ŋ	17		i	17	
—	18	d	v	18	d	ŋ	18		i	18	
d	19	d	v	19	d	ŋ	19		i	19	
d	20	d	v	20	d	ŋ	20		i	20	
d	21	d	v	21	d	ŋ	21		i	21	
d	22	d	v	22	d	ŋ	22		i	22	
d	23		v	23		ŋ	23		i	23	
d	24		v	24		ŋ	24		i	24	

Test phoneme /u/			Test phoneme /ɔ/			Test phoneme /w/			Test phoneme /h/		
Arresting position		Releasing position	Arresting position		Releasing position	Arresting position		Releasing position	Arresting position		Releasing position
u	1		ɔ	1			1	w		1	h
u	2		ɔ	2			2	w		2	h
u	3		ɔ	3			3	w		3	h
u	4		ɔ	4			4	w		4	h
u	5		ɔ	5			5	w		5	h
u	6		ɔ	6			6	w		6	h
u	7		ɔ	7			7	w		7	h

Test phoneme /u/		Test phoneme /ɔ/		Test phoneme /w/		Test phoneme /h/	
Arresting position	Releasing position	Arresting position	Releasing position	Arresting position	Releasing position	Arresting position	Releasing position
u	8	ɔ	8	8	w	8	h
u	9	ɔ	9	9	w	9	h
u	10	ɔ	10	10	w	10	h
u	11	ɔ	11	11	w	11	h
u	12	ɔ	12	12	w	12	h
u	13	ɔ	13	13	w	13	h
u	14	ɔ	14	14	w	14	h
u	15	ɔ	15	15	w	15	h
u	16	ɔ	16	16	w	16	h
u	17	ɔ	17	17	w	17	h
u	18	ɔ	18	18	w	18	h
u	19	ɔ	19	19	w	19	h
u	20	ɔ	20	20	w	20	h
u	21	ɔ	21	21	w	21	h
u	22	ɔ	22	22	w	22	h
u	23	ɔ	23	23	w	23	h
u	24	ɔ	24	24	w	24	h

Test phoneme /ɪ/		Test phoneme /ɛ/		Test phoneme /æ/		Test phoneme /ʌ/	
Arresting position	Releasing position	Arresting position	Releasing position	Arresting position	Releasing position	Arresting position	Releasing position
1	ɪ	1	ɛ	1	æ	1	ʌ
2	ɪ	2	ɛ	2	æ	2	ʌ
3	ɪ	3	ɛ	3	æ	3	ʌ
4	ɪ	4	ɛ	4	æ	4	ʌ
5	ɪ	5	ɛ	5	æ	5	ʌ
6	ɪ	6	ɛ	6	æ	6	ʌ
7	ɪ	7	ɛ	7	æ	7	ʌ
8	ɪ	8	ɛ	8	æ	8	ʌ
9	ɪ	9	ɛ	9	æ	9	ʌ
10	ɪ	10	ɛ	10	æ	10	ʌ
11	ɪ	11	ɛ	11	æ	11	ʌ
12	ɪ	12	ɛ	12	æ	12	ʌ
13	ɪ	13	ɛ	13	æ	13	ʌ
14	ɪ	14	ɛ	14	æ	14	ʌ
15	ɪ	15	ɛ	15	æ	15	ʌ
16	ɪ	16	ɛ	16	æ	16	ʌ
17	ɪ	17	ɛ	17	æ	17	ʌ
18	ɪ	18	ɛ	18	æ	18	ʌ
19	ɪ	19	ɛ	19	æ	19	ʌ
20	ɪ	20	ɛ	20	æ	20	ʌ

Test phoneme /ɪ/			Test phoneme /ɛ/			Test phoneme /æ/			Test phoneme /ʌ/		
Arresting position		Releasing position	Arresting position		Releasing position	Arresting position		Releasing position	Arresting position		Releasing position
	21	ɪ		21	ɛ		21	æ		21	ʌ
	22	ɪ		22	ɛ		22	æ		22	ʌ
	23			23			23			23	
	24			24			24			24	

EXERCISES

A. List the number of times the phoneme /p/ was tested on the McDonald Deep Test for Child 1.
B. What phonemes did the child substitute for /t/?
C. Which features differentiate the substitution phonemes of /θ/ and /ð/ from the target phoneme /s/?
D. On which features do the /b/ and /m/ substitutions differ from the test phoneme /v/?

ANSWERS TO EXERCISES

A. The /p/ was tested 46 times on the McDonald: 24 times in the arresting position and 22 times in the releasing position.
B. The child substituted /d/ for /t/ and /k/ for /t/.
C. The /θ/ differs from /s/ on the strident feature. The /ð/ differs from /s/ on the voicing and strident features.
D. The /v/ differs from /b/ on the continuant and strident features. The /v/ differs from /m/ on the continuant, nasal, and strident features.

10

Distinctive Feature Analysis Worksheet

A sample of the worksheet used in the distinctive feature analysis is presented in Table 4. Both correct responses and substitution responses from the articulation sample are transferred to this worksheet. Features of each test phoneme and substitution are recorded and analyzed for correct feature usage. An individual worksheet is prepared for each phoneme that is tested. The test phoneme should be specified at the top of each worksheet along with the total number of times the phoneme is sampled.

The worksheet is divided into four columns. The first column is labeled "Test Phoneme and Number of Times Correct." The phoneme that is tested is written under this heading. Beneath that, the number of times the child produced the phoneme correctly is specified. For example, in completing a worksheet for the first phoneme tested for Child 1, the /p/ is written beneath the heading. Under the /p/ the number "10" is recorded since /p/ was produced correctly 10 times on the articulation test.

The second column on the worksheet is for listing any substitution that occurred for the test phoneme and the number of times each substitution occurred. This column is headed "Phonemes Substituted and Number of Occurrences." Continuing the worksheet of Child 1 for /p/, the /b/ was produced 36 times when /p/ was tested. Therefore, /b/ is placed in this column along with the number "36" for the number of occurrences.

The third column on the worksheet is entitled "Number of Omissions." In this column, the number of times the child omits the test phoneme is specified. For Child 1, the test phoneme /p/ was never omitted; so the number "0" is recorded.

The last column headed "Number of Times Features Used Correctly" refers to the 13 rows on the left of the worksheet where the 13 distinctive features are listed. Across from each feature, the (+) or (−) feature aspect is entered for the test phoneme and for each substituted phoneme. Using Table 2, the (+) and (−) aspects are marked under the respective vertical columns for "Test Phoneme" and "Substitution Phonemes." For Child 1, the column for the test phoneme and the column for the substitution phoneme /b/ would be marked as follows:

	Test phoneme	Substitution
	p (10)	b (36)
Vocalic	−	−
Consonantal	+	+
High	−	−

Table 4. Distinctive feature analysis worksheet

Test phoneme ________

	Test phoneme and number of times correct	Phonemes substituted and number of occurrences	Number of omissions	Number of times features used correctly
	____ ____	____ ____ ____ ____ ____ ____	____	____ ____
Vocalic				
Consonantal				
High				
Back				
Low				
Anterior				
Coronal				
Round				
Tense				
Voice				
Continuant				
Nasal				
Strident				

(Additional copies of this analysis worksheet can be found at the back of the book.)

Table 5. Completed worksheet of the phoneme /p/ for Child 1

Test phoneme /p/ (46 samples)				
	Test phoneme and number of times correct	Phonemes substituted and number of occurrences	Number of omissions	Number of times features used correctly
	p (10)	b (36)	(0)	
Vocalic	–	–		46
Consonantal	+	+		46
High	–	–		46
Back	–	–		46
Low	–	–		46
Anterior	+	+		46
Coronal	–	–		46
Round				
Tense				
Voice	–	+		10
Continuant	–	–		46
Nasal	–	–		46
Strident	–	–		46

	Test phoneme	Substitution
	p (10)	b (36)
Back	–	–
Low	–	–
Anterior	+	+
Coronal	–	–
Round		
Tense		
Voice	–	+
Continuant	–	–
Nasal	–	–
Strident	–	–

The number of times each feature aspect is produced correctly when the test phoneme is tested is entered in the last column "Number of Times Features Used Correctly." The total correct score for each feature is shown here after the numbers are added across the columns for the test phoneme and substitutions. If the (+) or (–) aspect of a feature in a substituted phoneme is the same as the feature aspect in the test phoneme, the number of times it occurred in the substitution is added to the number of times it occurred in the test phoneme to provide a total for the feature. For instance, Child 1 produced both the correct /p/ phoneme and the substituted phoneme /b/ when /p/ was tested. The number of occurrences for /p/ is 10 and for /b/, 36. Both /p/ and /b/ are (–) vocalic. Therefore, the total number of times the (–) vocalic feature was correct when /p/ was tested is 46. Both /p/ and /b/ are (+) consonantal. The total for (+) consonantal would also be 46. The test phoneme /p/ differs from the /b/ substitution in the voicing feature. For this feature aspect, the number of occurrences of /b/ cannot be added to those for /p/. The total for (–) voicing when /p/ is the test phoneme is therefore only 10. The occurrence of (+) voicing for /b/ cannot be added to the total because /b/ is (+) voice and /p/ is (–) voice. The (+) or (–) aspect of a feature in a substitution can be included in the total only if it matches the (+) or (–) aspect of the feature of the test phoneme. A completed worksheet for /p/ for Child 1 is presented in Table 5.

EXERCISES

A. Complete a separate worksheet for all phonemes on which Child 1 was tested.

ANSWER TO EXERCISE A, DISTINCTIVE FEATURE WORKSHEET, CHILD 1

	Test phoneme and number of times correct	Phonemes substituted and number of occurrences	Number of omissions	Number of times features used correctly
	p (10)	b (36)		
Vocalic	–	–		46
Consonantal	+	+		46
High	–	–		46
Back	–	–		46
Low	–	–		46
Anterior	+	+		46
Coronal	–	–		46
Round				

	Test phoneme and number of times correct	Phonemes substituted and number of occurrences		Number of omissions	Number of times features used correctly
	p (10)	b (36)			
Tense					
Voice	–	+			10
Continuant	–	–			46
Nasal	–	–			46
Strident	–	–			46
	t (13)	d (15)	k (13)	(5)	
Vocalic	–	–	–		41
Consonantal	+	+	+		41
High	–	–	+		28
Back	–	–	+		28
Low	–	–	–		41
Anterior	+	+	–		28
Coronal	+	+	–		28
Round					
Tense					
Voice	–	+	–		26
Continuant	–	–	–		41
Nasal	–	–	–		41
Strident	–	–	–		41
	s (0)	θ (22)	ð (19)	(5)	
Vocalic	–	–	–		41
Consonantal	+	+	+		41
High	–	–	–		41
Back	–	–	–		41
Low	–	–	–		41
Anterior	+	+	+		41
Coronal	+	+	+		41
Round					
Tense					
Voice	–	–	+		22
Continuant	+	+	+		41
Nasal	–	–	–		41
Strident	+	–	–		0

	Test phoneme and number of times correct	Phonemes substituted and number of occurrences		Number of omissions	Number of times features used correctly
	v (0)	b (39)	m (5)	(2)	
Vocalic	–	–	–		44
Consonantal	+	+	+		44
High	–	–	–		44
Back	–	–	–		44
Low	–	–	–		44
Anterior	+	+	+		44
Coronal	–	–	–		44
Round					
Tense					
Voice	+	+	+		44
Continuant	+	–	–		0
Nasal	–	–	+		39
Strident	+	–	–		0
	b (46)				
Vocalic	–				46
Consonantal	+				46
High	–				46
Back	–				46
Low	–				46
Anterior	+				46
Coronal	–				46
Round					
Tense					
Voice	+				46
Continuant	–				46
Nasal	–				46
Strident	–				46
	d (46)				
Vocalic	–				46
Consonantal	+				46
High	–				46
Back	–				46
Low	–				46
Anterior	+				46

	Test phoneme and number of times correct	Phonemes substituted and number of occurrences	Number of omissions	Number of times features used correctly
	d (46)			
Coronal	+			46
Round				
Tense				
Voice	+			46
Continuant	–			46
Nasal	–			46
Strident	–			46
	k (24)	d (22)		
Vocalic	–	–		46
Consonantal	+	+		46
High	+	–		24
Back	+	–		24
Low	–	–		46
Anterior	–	+		24
Coronal	–	+		24
Round				
Tense				
Voice	–	+		24
Continuant	–	–		46
Nasal	–	–		46
Strident	–	–		46
	g (24)	d (22)		
Vocalic	–	–		46
Consonantal	+	+		46
High	+	–		24
Back	+	–		24
Low	–	–		46
Anterior	–	+		24
Coronal	–	+		24
Round				
Tense				
Voice	+	+		46
Continuant	–	–		46
Nasal	–	–		46
Strident	–	–		46

	Test phoneme and number of times correct	Phonemes substituted and number of occurrences	Number of omissions	Number of times features used correctly
	m (46)			
Vocalic	–			46
Consonantal	+			46
High	–			46
Back	–			46
Low	–			46
Anterior	+			46
Coronal	–			46
Round				
Tense				
Voice	+			46
Continuant	–			46
Nasal	+			46
Strident	–			46
	n (46)			
Vocalic	–			46
Consonantal	+			46
High	–			46
Back	–			46
Low	–			46
Anterior	+			46
Coronal	+			46
Round				
Tense				
Voice	+			46
Continuant	–			46
Nasal	+			46
Strident	–			46
	l (25)		(21)	
Vocalic	+			25
Consonantal	+			25
High	–			25
Back	–			25
Low	–			25
Anterior	+			25

	Test phoneme and number of times correct	Phonemes substituted and number of occurrences		Number of omissions	Number of times features used correctly
	l (25)			(21)	
Coronal	+				25
Round					
Tense					
Voice	+				25
Continuant	+				25
Nasal	–				25
Strident	–				25
	r (0)	w (22)		(24)	
Vocalic	+	–			0
Consonantal	+	–			0
High	–	+			0
Back	–	+			0
Low	–	–			22
Anterior	–	–			22
Coronal	+	–			0
Round		+			
Tense		–			
Voice	+				0
Continuant	+				0
Nasal	–				0
Strident	–				0
	f (0)	v (24)	w (22)		
Vocalic	–	–	–		46
Consonantal	+	+	–		24
High	–	–	+		24
Back	–	–	+		24
Low	–	–	–		46
Anterior	+	+	–		24
Coronal	–	–	–		46
Round			+		
Tense			–		
Voice	–	+			0
Continuant	+	+			24
Nasal	–	–			24
Strident	+	+			24

	Test phoneme and number of times correct	Phonemes substituted and number of occurrences			Number of omissions	Number of times features used correctly
	θ (0)	t (9)	d (37)			
Vocalic	–	–	–			46
Consonantal	+	+	+			46
High	–	–	–			46
Back	–	–	–			46
Low	–	–	–			46
Anterior	+	+	+			46
Coronal	+	+	+			46
Round						
Tense						
Voice	–	–	+			9
Continuant	+	–	–			0
Nasal	–	–	–			46
Strident	–	–	–			46
	z (0)	d (38)			(8)	
Vocalic	–	–				38
Consonantal	+	+				38
High	–	–				38
Back	–	–				38
Low	–	–				38
Anterior	+	+				38
Coronal	+	+				38
Round						
Tense						
Voice	+	+				38
Continuant	+	–				0
Nasal	–	–				38
Strident	+	–				0
	ʃ (0)	t (3)	d (18)	g (20)	(5)	
Vocalic	–	–	–	–		41
Consonantal	+	+	+	+		41
High	+	–	–	+		20
Back	–	–	–	+		21
Low	–	–	–	–		41
Anterior	–	+	+	–		20

	Test phoneme and number of times correct	Phonemes substituted and number of occurrences			Number of omissions	Number of times features used correctly
Coronal	+	+	+	−		21
Round						
Tense						
Voice	−	−	+	+		3
Continuant	+	−	−	−		0
Nasal	−	−	−	−		41
Strident	+	−	−	−		0
	tʃ (0)	d (33)			(13)	
Vocalic	−	−				33
Consonantal	+	+				33
High	+	−				0
Back	−	−				33
Low	−	−				33
Anterior	−	+				0
Coronal	+	+				33
Round						
Tense						
Voice	−	+				0
Continuant	−	−				33
Nasal	−	−				33
Strident	+	−				0
	dʒ (0)	d (22)	v (24)			
Vocalic	−	−	−			46
Consonantal	+	+	+			46
High	+	−	−			0
Back	−	−	−			46
Low	−	−	−			46
Anterior	−	+	+			0
Coronal	+	+	−			22
Round						
Tense						
Voice	+	+	+			46
Continuant	−	−	+			22
Nasal	−	−	−			46
Strident	+	−	+			24

	Test phoneme and number of times correct	Phonemes substituted and number of occurrences	Number of omissions	Number of times features used correctly
	ŋ (24)			
Vocalic	–			24
Consonantal	+			24
High	+			24
Back	+			24
Low	–			24
Anterior	–			24
Coronal	–			24
Round				
Tense				
Voice	+			24
Continuant	–			24
Nasal	+			24
Strident	–			24
	i (24)			
Vocalic	+			24
Consonantal	–			24
High	+			24
Back	–			24
Low	–			24
Anterior	–			24
Coronal	–			24
Round	–			24
Tense	+			24
Voice				
Continuant				
Nasal				
Strident				
	u (24)			
Vocalic	+			24
Consonantal	–			24
High	+			24
Back	+			24
Low	–			24
Anterior	–			24

	Test phoneme and number of times correct	Phonemes substituted and number of occurrences	Number of omissions	Number of times features used correctly
	u (24)			
Coronal	–			24
Round	+			24
Tense	+			24
Voice				
Continuant				
Nasal				
Strident				
	ɔ (24)			
Vocalic	+			24
Consonantal	–			24
High	–			24
Back	+			24
Low	+			24
Anterior	–			24
Coronal	–			24
Round	+			24
Tense	–			24
Voice				
Continuant				
Nasal				
Strident				
	w (22)			
Vocalic	–			22
Consonantal	–			22
High	+			22
Back	+			22
Low	–			22
Anterior	–			22
Coronal	–			22
Round	+			22
Tense	–			22
Voice				
Continuant				
Nasal				
Strident				

	Test phoneme and number of times correct	Phonemes substituted and number of occurrences	Number of omissions	Number of times features used correctly
	h (22)			
Vocalic	–			22
Consonantal	–			22
High	–			22
Back	–			22
Low	+			22
Anterior	–			22
Coronal	–			22
Round				
Tense				
Voice	–			22
Continuant	+			22
Nasal	–			22
Strident	–			22
	ɪ (22)			
Vocalic	+			22
Consonantal	–			22
High	+			22
Back	–			22
Low	–			22
Anterior	–			22
Coronal	–			22
Round	–			22
Tense	–			22
Voice				
Continuant				
Nasal				
Strident				
	ϵ (22)			
Vocalic	+			22
Consonantal	–			22
High	–			22
Back	–			22
Low	–			22
Anterior	–			22

	Test phoneme and number of times correct	Phonemes substituted and number of occurrences	Number of omissions	Number of times features used correctly
Coronal	–			22
Round	–			22
Tense	–			22
Voice				
Continuant				
Nasal				
Strident				
	æ (22)			
Vocalic	+			22
Consonantal	–			22
High	–			22
Back	–			22
Low	+			22
Anterior	–			22
Coronal	–			22
Round	–			22
Tense	–			22
Voice				
Continuant				
Nasal				
Strident				
	ʌ (22)			
Vocalic	+			22
Consonantal	–			22
High	–			22
Back	+			22
Low	–			22
Anterior	–			22
Coronal	–			22
Round	–			22
Tense	–			22
Voice				
Continuant				
Nasal				
Strident				

11

Distinctive Feature Analysis Sheet

Completion of an analysis sheet is the last step. A sample of the analysis sheet is presented in Table 6. The purpose of this part of the analysis is to compute, across all phonemes tested, the percentage at which each feature is incorrect in the child's repertoire. The total scores from the worksheet for each feature of each phoneme are transferred to the analysis sheet in this final computation. A separate analysis sheet is completed for each of the 13 distinctive features. Each sheet has two sections: the left section is for the (+) aspect of a feature and the right section is for the (−) aspect.

Table 6. Distinctive feature analysis sheet

Analysis sheet for (+) and (−) ______ contrasts					
(+) ______ Feature			(−) ______ Feature		
Phoneme in which feature is present	Number of possible occurrences	Number of correct occurrences	Phoneme in which feature is present	Number of possible occurrences	Number of correct occurrences
	Total = ______	Total = ______		Total = ______	Total = ______
	% Incorrect = ______			% Incorrect = ______	

(Additional copies of this analysis sheet can be found at the back of the book.)

The first column in each section is labeled "Phoneme in Which Feature is Present." In this column, each test phoneme containing that aspect of a feature is listed. For example, an analysis sheet of the continuant feature for Child 1 shows the following phonemes listed in each section.

(+) Continuant feature	(–) Continuant feature
f	p
v	b
θ	t
s	d
z	k
l	m
r	n
h	tʃ
ʃ	dʒ
	g
	ŋ

The second column on the analysis sheet is "Number of Possible Occurrences." In this column, the total number of times the feature could have been produced correctly when each phoneme was tested is entered. Stated another way, this is the total number of times that particular phoneme was sampled on the articulation test. For example, (+) continuancy could have been produced correctly 46 times when /f/ was tested. Completing this column for Child 1 shows 46 possible occurrences of (+) and (–) continuancy for most phonemes. However, (+) and (–) continuancy could not occur as frequently when /h/ and /ŋ/ were tested because of the smaller sample size for those two phonemes.

The last column on the analysis sheet is labeled "Number of Correct Occurrences." The number to be entered in this column is transferred from the completed worksheets for each phoneme. The number to be transferred is the total score of correct feature production for each test phoneme and is found in the final column of each worksheet labeled "Number of Times Each Feature Used Correctly." For instance, when the /v/ was tested for Child 1, the (+) continuant feature was never produced correctly. On the other hand, (–) continuancy was produced correctly 46 and 41 times in the contexts of the phonemes /p/ and /t/, respectively.

Completing the analysis sheet requires totaling the numbers in the columns "Number of Possible Occurrences" and "Number of Correct Occurrences" for both feature

(+) Continuant feature		(–) Continuant feature	
Phoneme in which feature is present	Number of possible occurrences	Phoneme in which feature is present	Number of possible occurrences
f	46	p	46
v	46	b	46
θ	46	t	46
s	46	d	46
z	46	k	46
l	46	m	46
r	46	n	46
h	22	tʃ	46
ʃ	46	dʒ	46
		g	46
		ŋ	24

aspects. The total for "Number of Correct Occurrences" is then divided by the total for "Number of Possible Occurrences." This results in a percentage of correct feature production. To compute the per cent incorrect, subtract the dividend from 100. A completed analysis sheet for the continuancy feature for Child 1 is presented in Table 7. Each per cent incorrect figure for the (+) and (−) aspects of each of the 13 distinctive features together provide a profile of a child's distinctive feature development and usage.

Table 7. Completed analysis sheet of the continuancy feature for Child 1

Analysis sheet for (+) and (−) continuant contrasts					
(+) Continuant feature			(−) Continuant feature		
Phoneme in which feature is present	Number of possible occurrences	Number of correct occurrences	Phoneme in which feature is present	Number of possible occurrences	Number of correct occurrences
f	46	24	p	46	46
v	46	0	b	46	46
θ	46	0	t	46	41
s	46	41	d	46	46
z	46	0	k	46	46
l	46	25	m	46	46
r	46	0	n	46	46
h	22	22	tʃ	46	33
ʃ	46	0	dʒ	46	22
			g	46	46
			ŋ	24	24
	Total = 390 % Incorrect = 71.3	Total = 112		Total = 484 % Incorrect = 8.7	Total = 442

EXERCISES

A. Complete a separate analysis sheet for the remaining 12 distinctive features for Child 1 using all 28 phonemes that were tested.

B. To demonstrate the application of the distinctive feature analysis for analyzing a smaller articulation sample, a second child's (Child 2) articulation responses are presented in Table 8. In this sample, the articulation responses were again evoked using the McDonald Deep Test of Articulation. However, only the first 10 items in the arresting position and the first 10 items in the releasing position are presented in the sample. Since most articulation errors involve only consonants, no responses to vowels are provided in the sample.

Complete a worksheet for each phoneme tested on the McDonald Deep Test of Articulation for Child 2.

C. Complete an analysis for all 13 distinctive features for Child 2.

Table 8. Articulation test responses from the McDonald Deep Test of Articulation for Child 2

Test phoneme /p/			Test phoneme /b/			Test phoneme /t/			Test phoneme /d/		
Arresting position		Releasing position	Arresting position		Releasing position	Arresting position		Releasing position	Arresting position		Releasing position
–	1	b	–	1	b	–	1	d	–	1	d
–	2	b	–	2	b	–	2	d	–	2	d
–	3	b	–	3	b	–	3	d	–	3	d
–	4	b	–	4	b	–	4	d	–	4	d
–	5	b	–	5	b	–	5	d	–	5	d
–	6	b	–	6	b	–	6	d	–	6	d
–	7	b	–	7	b	–	7	d	–	7	d
–	8	b	–	8	b	–	8	d	–	8	d
–	9	b	–	9	b	–	9	d	–	9	d
–	10	b	–	10	b	–	10	d	–	10	d

Test phoneme /k/			Test phoneme /g/			Test phoneme /m/			Test phoneme /n/		
Arresting position		Releasing position	Arresting position		Releasing position	Arresting position		Releasing position	Arresting position		Releasing position
–	1	d	–	1	d	n	1	m	n	1	n
–	2	d	–	2	d	n	2	m	n	2	n
–	3	d	–	3	d	n	3	m	n	3	n
–	4	d	–	4	d	n	4	m	n	4	n
–	5	d	–	5	d	n	5	m	n	5	n
–	6	d	–	6	d	n	6	m	n	6	n
–	7	d	–	7	d	n	7	m	n	7	n
–	8	d	–	8	d	n	8	m	n	8	n
–	9	d	–	9	d	n	9	m	n	9	n
–	10	d	–	10	d	n	10	m	n	10	n

Test phoneme /f/			Test phoneme /v/			Test phoneme /θ/			Test phoneme /s/		
Arresting position		Releasing position	Arresting position		Releasing position	Arresting position		Releasing position	Arresting position		Releasing position
–	1	b	–	1	b	–	1	d	–	1	d
–	2	b	–	2	b	–	2	d	–	2	d
–	3	b	–	3	b	–	3	d	–	3	d
–	4	b	–	4	b	–	4	d	–	4	d
–	5	b	–	5	b	–	5	d	–	5	d
–	6	b	–	6	b	–	6	d	–	6	d
–	7	b	–	7	b	–	7	d	–	7	d
–	8	b	–	8	b	–	8	d	–	8	d
–	9	b	–	9	b	–	9	d	–	9	d
–	10	b	–	10	b	–	10	d	–	10	d

Test phoneme /z/			Test phoneme /ʃ/			Test phoneme /tʃ/			Test phoneme /dʒ/		
Arresting position		Releasing position	Arresting position		Releasing position	Arresting position		Releasing position	Arresting position		Releasing position
—	1	dʒ	—	1	dʒ	—	1	dʒ	—	1	d
—	2	—	—	2	dʒ	—	2	dʒ	—	2	d
—	3	dʒ	—	3	ʃ	—	3	dʒ	—	3	d
—	4	dʒ	—	4	—	—	4	dʒ	—	4	d
—	5	—	—	5	t	—	5	tʃ	—	5	d
—	6	d	—	6	t	—	6	dʒ	—	6	d
—	7	d	—	7	d	—	7	dʒ	—	7	d
—	8	d	—	8	dʒ	—	8	—	—	8	d
—	9	—	—	9	t	—	9	tʃ	—	9	d
—	10	—	—	10	d	—	10	dʒ	—	10	d

Test phoneme /l/			Test phoneme /r/			Test phoneme /ŋ/		
Arresting position		Releasing position	Arresting position		Releasing position	Arresting position		Releasing position
—	1	—	r	1	w	ŋ	1	
—	2	—	r	2	w	ŋ	2	
—	3	—	r	3	w	ŋ	3	
—	4	—	r	4	w	ŋ	4	
—	5	—	r	5	w	ŋ	5	
—	6	—	r	6	w	ŋ	6	
—	7	—	r	7	w	ŋ	7	
—	8	n	r	8	w	ŋ	8	
—	9	n	r	9	w	ŋ	9	
—	10	n	r	10	w	ŋ	10	

ANSWERS TO EXERCISE A, CHILD 1

Analysis sheet for (+) and (–) vocal contrasts					
(+) Vocalic feature			(–) Vocalic feature		
Phoneme in which feature is present	Number of possible occurrences	Number of correct occurrences	Phoneme in which feature is present	Number of possible occurrences	Number of correct occurrences
l	46	25	p	46	46
r	46	0	b	46	46
i	24	24	t	46	41
ɪ	22	22	d	46	46
ɛ	22	22	f	46	46
æ	22	22	v	46	44
ʌ	22	22	θ	46	46
u	24	24	s	46	41
ɔ	24	24	z	46	38
			k	46	46
			g	46	46
			m	46	46
			n	46	46
			ŋ	24	24
			ʃ	46	41
			tʃ	46	33
			dʒ	46	46
			w	22	22
			h	22	22
	Total = 252	Total = 185		Total = 804	Total = 766
	% Incorrect = 26.6			% Incorrect = 4.8	

Analysis sheet for (+) and (−) consonantal contrasts					
(+) Consonantal feature			(−) Consonantal feature		
Phoneme in which feature is present	Number of possible occurrences	Number of correct occurrences	Phoneme in which feature is present	Number of possible occurrences	Number of correct occurrences
p	46	46	w	22	22
b	46	46	h	22	22
t	46	41	i	24	24
d	46	46	ɪ	22	22
f	46	24	ϵ	22	22
v	46	44	æ	22	22
θ	46	46	u	24	24
s	46	41	ɔ	24	24
k	46	46			
m	46	46			
n	46	46			
l	46	25			
r	46	0			
tʃ	46	33			
dʒ	46	46			
z	46	38			
ʃ	46	41			
g	46	46			
ŋ	24	24			
% Incorrect = 15	Total = 852	Total = 725	% Incorrect = 0	Total = 204	Total = 204

Analysis sheet for (+) and (–) high contrasts

(+) High feature			(–) High feature		
Phoneme in which feature is present	Number of possible occurrences	Number of correct occurrences	Phoneme in which feature is present	Number of possible occurrences	Number of correct occurrences
k	46	24	p	46	46
w	22	22	b	46	46
tʃ	46	0	t	46	28
dʒ	46	0	d	46	46
ʃ	46	20	f	46	24
g	46	24	v	46	44
ŋ	24	24	θ	46	46
i	24	24	s	46	41
ɪ	22	22	m	46	46
u	24	24	n	46	46
			l	46	25
			r	46	0
			h	22	22
			z	46	38
			ɛ	22	22
			æ	22	22
			ʌ	22	22
			ɔ	24	24
	Total = 346	Total = 184		Total = 710	Total = 588
	% Incorrect = 46.9			% Incorrect = 17.2	

Analysis sheet for (+) and (−) back contrasts					
(+) Back feature			(−) Back feature		
Phoneme in which feature is present	Number of possible occurrences	Number of correct occurrences	Phoneme in which feature is present	Number of possible occurrences	Number of correct occurrences
k	46	24	p	46	46
w	22	22	b	46	46
g	46	24	t	46	28
ŋ	24	24	d	46	46
ʌ	22	22	f	46	24
u	24	24	v	46	44
ɔ	24	24	θ	46	46
			s	46	41
			m	46	46
			n	46	46
			l	46	25
			r	46	0
			h	22	22
			tʃ	46	33
			dʒ	46	46
			ʃ	46	21
			z	46	38
			i	24	24
			ɪ	22	22
			ϵ	22	22
			æ	22	22
	Total = 208	**Total = 164**		Total = 848	**Total = 688**
% Incorrect = 21.2			% Incorrect = 18.9		

Analysis sheet for (+) and (−) low contrasts

(+) Low feature			(−) Low feature		
Phoneme in which feature is present	Number of possible occurrences	Number of correct occurrences	Phoneme in which feature is present	Number of possible occurrences	Number of correct occurrences
h	22	22	p	46	46
æ	22	22	b	46	46
ɔ	24	24	t	46	41
			d	46	46
			f	46	46
			v	46	44
			θ	46	46
			s	46	41
			k	46	46
			m	46	46
			n	46	46
			l	46	25
			r	46	22
			w	22	22
			tʃ	46	33
			dʒ	46	46
			z	46	38
			ʃ	46	41
			g	46	46
			ŋ	24	24
			i	24	24
			ɪ	22	22
			ϵ	22	22
			ʌ	22	22
			u	24	24
	Total = 68 % Incorrect = 0	**Total = 68**		Total = 988 % Incorrect = 8.5	**Total = 905**

Analysis sheet for (+) and (−) anterior contrasts

(+) Anterior feature			(−) Anterior feature		
Phoneme in which feature is present	Number of possible occurrences	Number of correct occurrences	Phoneme in which feature is present	Number of possible occurrences	Number of correct occurrences
p	46	46	k	46	24
b	46	46	r	46	22
t	46	28	w	22	22
d	46	46	h	22	22
f	46	24	tʃ	46	0
v	46	44	dʒ	46	0
θ	46	46	ʃ	46	20
s	46	41	g	46	24
m	46	46	ŋ	24	24
n	46	46	i	24	24
l	46	25	ɪ	22	22
z	46	38	ɛ	22	22
			æ	22	22
			ʌ	22	22
			u	24	24
			ɔ	24	24
	Total = 552 % Incorrect = 13.8	**Total = 476**		Total = 504 % Incorrect = 37	**Total = 318**

Analysis sheet for (+) and (−) coronal contrasts

(+) Coronal feature			(−) Coronal feature		
Phoneme in which feature is present	Number of possible occurrences	Number of correct occurrences	Phoneme in which feature is present	Number of possible occurrences	Number of correct occurrences
t	46	28	p	46	46
d	46	46	b	46	46
θ	46	46	f	46	46
s	46	41	v	46	44
n	46	46	k	46	24
l	46	25	m	46	46
r	46	0	w	22	22
tʃ	46	33	h	22	22
dʒ	46	22	g	46	24
z	46	38	ŋ	24	24
ʃ	46	21	i	24	24
			ɪ	22	22
			ɛ	22	22
			æ	22	22
			ʌ	22	22
			ụ	24	24
			ɔ	24	24
% Incorrect = 31.7	Total = 506	Total = 346	% Incorrect = 8.4	Total = 550	Total = 504

Analysis sheet for (+) and (−) round contrasts					
(+) Round feature			(−) Round feature		
Phoneme in which feature is present	Number of possible occurrences	Number of correct occurrences	Phoneme in which feature is present	Number of possible occurrences	Number of correct occurrences
u	24	24	i	24	24
ɔ	24	24	ɪ	22	22
w	22	22	ɛ	22	22
			æ	22	22
			ʌ	22	22
% Incorrect = 0	Total = 70	Total = 70	% Incorrect = 0	Total = 112	Total = 112

Analysis sheet for (+) and (−) tense contrasts

(+) Tense feature			(−) Tense feature		
Phoneme in which feature is present	Number of possible occurrences	Number of correct occurrences	Phoneme in which feature is present	Number of possible occurrences	Number of correct occurrences
i	24	24	w	22	22
u	24	24	ɪ	22	22
			ɛ	22	22
			æ	22	22
			ʌ	22	22
			ɔ	24	24
	Total = 48 % Incorrect = 0	Total = 48		Total = 134 % Incorrect = 0	Total = 134

Analysis sheet for (+) and (−) voice contrasts

(+) Voice feature			(−) Voice feature		
Phoneme in which feature is present	Number of possible occurrences	Number of correct occurrences	Phoneme in which feature is present	Number of possible occurrences	Number of correct occurrences
b	46	46	p	46	10
d	46	46	t	46	26
v	46	44	f	46	0
m	46	46	θ	46	9
n	46	46	s	46	22
l	46	25	k	46	24
r	46	0	h	22	22
dʒ	46	46	tʃ	46	0
z	46	38	ʃ	46	3
g	46	46			
ŋ	24	24			
	Total = 484	Total = 407		Total = 390	Total = 116
% Incorrect = 15.9			% Incorrect = 70.3		

Analysis sheet for (+) and (−) nasal contrasts

(+) Nasal feature			(−) Nasal feature		
Phoneme in which feature is present	Number of possible occurrences	Number of correct occurrences	Phoneme in which feature is present	Number of possible occurrences	Number of correct occurrences
m	46	46	p	46	46
n	46	46	b	46	46
ŋ	24	24	t	46	41
			d	46	46
			f	46	24
			v	46	39
			θ	46	46
			s	46	41
			k	46	46
			l	46	25
			r	46	0
			h	22	22
			tʃ	46	33
			dʒ	46	46
			z	46	38
			ʃ	46	41
			g	46	46
	Total = 116	Total = 116		Total = 758	Total = 626
% Incorrect = 0			% Incorrect = 17.5		

Analysis sheet for (+) and (−) strident contrasts

(+) Strident feature			(−) Strident feature		
Phoneme in which feature is present	Number of possible occurrences	Number of correct occurrences	Phoneme in which feature is present	Number of possible occurrences	Number of correct occurrences
f	46	24	p	46	46
v	46	0	b	46	46
s	46	0	t	46	41
tʃ	46	0	d	46	46
dʒ	46	24	θ	46	46
z	46	0	k	46	46
ʃ	46	0	m	46	46
			n	46	46
			l	46	25
			r	46	0
			h	22	22
			g	46	46
			ŋ	24	24
	Total = 322	Total = 48		Total = 552	Total = 480
	% Incorrect = 85.1			% Incorrect = 13	

ANSWERS TO EXERCISE B, CHILD 2

	Test phoneme and number of times correct	Phonemes substituted and number of occurrences	Number of omissions	Number of times features used correctly
	p (0)	b (10)	(10)	
Vocalic	–	–		10
Consonantal	+	+		10
High	–	–		10
Back	–	–		10
Low	–	–		10
Anterior	+	+		10
Coronal	–	–		10
Round				
Tense				
Voice	–	+		0
Continuant	–	–		10
Nasal	–	–		10
Strident	–	–		10
	t (0)	d (10)		
Vocalic	–	–		10
Consonantal	+	+		10
High	–	–		10
Back	–	–		10
Low	–	–		10
Anterior	+	+		10
Coronal	+	+		10
Round				
Tense				
Voice	–	+		0
Continuant	–	–		10
Nasal	–	–		10
Strident	–	–		10
	s (0)	d (10)	(10)	
Vocalic	–	–		10
Consonantal	+	+		10
High	–	–		10
Back	–	–		10
Low	–	–		10
Anterior	+	+		10
Coronal	+	+		10

	Test phoneme and number of times correct	Phonemes substituted and number of occurrences	Number of omissions	Number of times features used correctly
	s (0)	d (10)	(10)	
Round				
Tense				
Voice	–	+		0
Continuant	+	–		0
Nasal	–	–		10
Strident	+	–		0
	v (0)	b (10)	(10)	
Vocalic	–	–		10
Consonantal	+	+		10
High	–	–		10
Back	–	–		10
Low	–	–		10
Anterior	+	+		10
Coronal	–	–		10
Round				
Tense				
Voice	+	+		10
Continuant	+	–		0
Nasal	–	–		10
Strident	+	–		0
	b (10)		(10)	
Vocalic	–			10
Consonantal	+			10
High	–			10
Back	–			10
Low	–			10
Anterior	+			10
Coronal	–			10
Round				
Tense				
Voice	+			10
Continuant	–			10
Nasal	–			10
Strident	–			10

	Test phoneme and number of times correct	Phonemes substituted and number of occurrences	Number of omissions	Number of times features used correctly
	d (10)		(10)	
Vocalic	–			10
Consonantal	+			10
High	–			10
Back	–			10
Low	–			10
Anterior	+			10
Coronal	+			10
Round				
Tense				
Voice	+			10
Continuant	–			10
Nasal	–			10
Strident	–			10
	k (0)	d (10)	(10)	
Vocalic	–	–		10
Consonantal	+	+		10
High	+	–		0
Back	+	–		0
Low	–	–		10
Anterior	–	+		0
Coronal	–	+		0
Round				
Tense				
Voice	–	+		0
Continuant	–	–		10
Nasal	–	–		10
Strident	–	–		10
	g (0)	d (10)	(10)	
Vocalic	–	–		10
Consonantal	+	+		10
High	+	–		0
Back	+	–		0
Low	–	–		10
Anterior	–	+		0

	Test phoneme and number of times correct	Phonemes substituted and number of occurrences	Number of omissions	Number of times features used correctly
	g (0)	d (10)	(10)	
Coronal	–	+		0
Round				
Tense				
Voice	+	+		10
Continuant	–	–		10
Nasal	–	–		10
Strident	–	–		10
	m (10)	n (10)		
Vocalic	–	–		20
Consonantal	+	+		20
High	–	–		20
Back	–	–		20
Low	–	–		20
Anterior	+	+		20
Coronal	–	+		10
Round				
Tense				
Voice	+	+		20
Continuant	–	–		20
Nasal	+	+		20
Strident	–	–		20
	n (20)			
Vocalic	–			20
Consonantal	+			20
High	–			20
Back	–			20
Low	–			20
Anterior	+			20
Coronal	+			20
Round				
Tense				
Voice	+			20
Continuant	–			20
Nasal	+			20
Strident	–			20

	Test phoneme and number of times correct	Phonemes substituted and number of occurrences	Number of omissions	Number of times features used correctly
	l (0)	n (3)	(17)	
Vocalic	+	–		0
Consonantal	+	+		3
High	–	–		3
Back	–	–		3
Low	–	–		3
Anterior	+	+		3
Coronal	+	+		3
Round				
Tense				
Voice	+	+		3
Continuant	+	–		0
Nasal	–	+		0
Strident	–	–		3
	r (10)	w (10)		
Vocalic	+	–		10
Consonantal	+	–		10
High	–	+		10
Back	–	+		10
Low	–	–		20
Anterior	–	–		20
Coronal	+	–		10
Round		+		
Tense		–		
Voice	+			10
Continuant	+			10
Nasal	–			10
Strident	–			10
	f (0)	b (10)	(10)	
Vocalic	–	–		10
Consonantal	+	+		10
High	–	–		10
Back	–	–		10
Low	–	–		10
Anterior	+	+		10
Coronal	–	–		10

	Test phoneme and number of times correct	Phonemes substituted and number of occurrences		Number of omissions	Number of times features used correctly
	f (0)	b (10)		(10)	
Round					
Tense					
Voice	–	+			0
Continuant	+	–			0
Nasal	–	–			10
Strident	+	–			0
	θ (0)	d (10)		(10)	
Vocalic	–	–			10
Consonantal	+	+			10
High	–	–			10
Back	–	–			10
Low	–	–			10
Anterior	+	+			10
Coronal	+	+			10
Round					
Tense					
Voice	–	+			0
Continuant	+	–			0
Nasal	–	–			10
Strident	–	–			10
	z (0)	dʒ (3)	d (3)	(14)	
Vocalic	–	–	–		6
Consonantal	+	+	+		6
High	–	+	–		3
Back	–	–	–		6
Low	–	–	–		6
Anterior	+	–	+		3
Coronal	+	+	+		6
Round					
Tense					
Voice	+	+	+		6
Continuant	+	–	–		0
Nasal	–	–	–		6
Strident	+	+	–		3

	Test phoneme and number of times correct	Phonemes substituted and number of occurrences			Number of omissions	Number of times features used correctly
	ʃ (1)	dʒ (3)	t (3)	d (2)	(11)	
Vocalic	–	–	–	–		9
Consonantal	+	+	+	+		9
High	+	+	–	–		4
Back	–	–	–	–		9
Low	–	–	–	–		9
Anterior	–	–	+	+		4
Coronal	+	+	+	+		9
Round						
Tense						
Voice	–	+	–	+		4
Continuant	+	–	–	–		1
Nasal	–	–	–	–		9
Strident	+	+	–	–		4
	tʃ (2)	dʒ (6)	d (1)	(11)		
Vocalic	–	–	–			9
Consonantal	+	+	+			9
High	+	+	–			8
Back	–	–	–			9
Low	–	–	–			9
Anterior	–	–	+			8
Coronal	+	+	+			9
Round						
Tense						
Voice	–	+	+			2
Continuant	–	–	–			9
Nasal	–	–	–			9
Strident	+	+	–			8
	dʒ (0)	d (10)			(10)	
Vocalic	–	–				10
Consonantal	+	+				10
High	+	–				0
Back	–	–				10
Low	–	–				10
Anterior	–	+				0
Coronal	+	+				10

	Test phoneme and number of times correct	Phonemes substituted and number of occurrences	Number of omissions	Number of times features used correctly
	dʒ (0)	d (10)	(10)	
Round				
Tense				
Voice	+	+		10
Continuant	−	−		10
Nasal	−	−		10
Strident	+	−		0
	ŋ (10)			
Vocalic	−			10
Consonantal	+			10
High	+			10
Back	+			10
Low	−			10
Anterior	−			10
Coronal	−			10
Round				
Tense				
Voice	+			10
Continuant	−			10
Nasal	+			10
Strident	−			10

ANSWERS TO EXERCISE C, CHILD 2

Analysis sheet for (+) and (−) vocalic contrasts

(+) Vocalic feature			(−) Vocalic feature		
Phoneme in which feature is present	Number of possible occurrences	Number of correct occurrences	Phoneme in which feature is present	Number of possible occurrences	Number of correct occurrences
l	20	0	p	20	10
r	20	10	b	20	10
			t	20	10
			d	20	10
			f	20	10
			v	20	10
			θ	20	10
			s	20	10
			z	20	6
			k	20	10
			g	20	10
			m	20	20
			n	20	20
			ŋ	10	10
			ʃ	20	9
			tʃ	20	9
			dʒ	20	10
	Total = 40	Total = 10		Total = 330	Total = 184
	% Incorrect = 75			% Incorrect = 44.2	

Analysis sheet for (+) and (–) consonantal contrasts

(+) Consonantal feature			(–) Consonantal feature		
Phoneme in which feature is present	Number of possible occurrences	Number of correct occurrences	Phoneme in which feature is present	Number of possible occurrences	Number of correct occurrences
p	20	10			
b	20	10			
t	20	10			
d	20	10			
f	20	10			
v	20	10			
θ	20	10			
s	20	10			
k	20	10			
m	20	20			
n	20	20			
l	20	3			
r	20	10			
tʃ	20	9			
dʒ	20	10			
z	20	6			
ʃ	20	9			
g	20	10			
ŋ	10	10			
	Total = 370	Total = 197		Total = ______	Total = ______
	% Incorrect = 46.8			% Incorrect = ______	

Analysis sheet for (+) and (−) high contrasts

(+) High feature			(−) High feature		
Phoneme in which feature is present	Number of possible occurrences	Number of correct occurrences	Phoneme in which feature is present	Number of possible occurrences	Number of correct occurrences
k	20	0	p	20	10
tʃ	20	8	b	20	10
dʒ	20	0	t	20	10
ʃ	20	4	d	20	10
g	20	0	f	20	10
ŋ	10	10	v	20	10
			θ	20	10
			s	20	10
			m	20	20
			n	20	20
			l	20	3
			r	20	10
			z	20	3
	Total = 110	Total = 22		Total = 260	Total = 136
	% Incorrect = 80			% Incorrect = 47.7	

Analysis sheet for (+) and (−) back contrasts					
(+) Back feature			(−) Back feature		
Phoneme in which feature is present	Number of possible occurrences	Number of correct occurrences	Phoneme in which feature is present	Number of possible occurrences	Number of correct occurrences
k	20	0	p	20	10
g	20	0	b	20	10
ŋ	10	10	t	20	10
			d	20	10
			f	20	10
			v	20	10
			θ	20	10
			s	20	10
			m	20	20
			n	20	20
			l	20	3
			r	20	10
			tʃ	20	9
			dʒ	20	10
			z	20	6
			ʃ	20	9
	Total = 50 % Incorrect = 80	Total = 10		Total = 320 % Incorrect = 47.8	Total = 167

Analysis sheet for (+) and (−) low contrasts

(+) Low feature			(−) Low feature		
Phoneme in which feature is present	Number of possible occurrences	Number of correct occurrences	Phoneme in which feature is present	Number of possible occurrences	Number of correct occurrences
			p	20	10
			b	20	10
			t	20	10
			d	20	10
			f	20	10
			v	20	10
			θ	20	10
			s	20	10
			k	20	10
			m	20	20
			n	20	20
			l	20	3
			r	20	20
			tʃ	20	9
			dʒ	20	10
			z	20	6
			ʃ	20	9
			g	20	10
			ŋ	10	10
	Total = ______	Total = _____		Total = 370	Total = 207
	% Incorrect = ______			% Incorrect = 44.1	

Analysis sheet for (+) and (−) anterior contrasts

(+) Anterior feature			(−) Anterior feature		
Phoneme in which feature is present	Number of possible occurrences	Number of correct occurrences	Phoneme in which feature is present	Number of possible occurrences	Number of correct occurrences
p	20	10	k	20	0
b	20	10	r	20	20
t	20	10	tʃ	20	8
d	20	10	dʒ	20	0
f	20	10	ʃ	20	4
v	20	10	g	20	0
θ	20	10	ŋ	10	10
s	20	10			
m	20	20			
n	20	20			
l	20	3			
z	20	3			
	Total = 240 % Incorrect = 47.5	Total = 126		Total = 130 % Incorrect = 67.7	Total = 42

Analysis sheet for (+) and (−) coronal contrasts

(+) Coronal feature			(−) Coronal feature		
Phoneme in which feature is present	Number of possible occurrences	Number of correct occurrences	Phoneme in which feature is present	Number of possible occurrences	Number of correct occurrences
t	20	10	p	20	10
d	20	10	b	20	10
θ	20	10	f	20	10
s	20	10	v	20	10
n	20	20	k	20	0
l	20	3	m	20	10
r	20	10	g	20	0
tʃ	20	9	ŋ	10	10
dʒ	20	10			
z	20	6			
ʃ	20	9			
	Total = 220	Total = 107		Total = 150	Total = 60
	% Incorrect = 51.4			% Incorrect = 60	

Analysis sheet for (+) and (−) voice contrasts					
(+) Voice feature			(−) Voice feature		
Phoneme in which feature is present	Number of possible occurrences	Number of correct occurrences	Phoneme in which feature is present	Number of possible occurrences	Number of correct occurrences
b	20	10	p	20	0
d	20	10	t	20	0
v	20	10	f	20	0
m	20	20	θ	20	0
n	20	20	s	20	0
l	20	3	k	20	0
r	20	10	tʃ	20	2
dʒ	20	10	ʃ	20	4
z	20	6			
g	20	10			
ŋ	10	10			
	Total = 210 % Incorrect = 43.3	Total = 119		Total = 160 % Incorrect = 96	Total = 6

Analysis sheet for (+) and (–) nasal contrasts

(+) Nasal feature			(–) Nasal feature		
Phoneme in which feature is present	Number of possible occurrences	Number of correct occurrences	Phoneme in which feature is present	Number of possible occurrences	Number of correct occurrences
m	20	20	p	20	10
n	20	20	b	20	10
ŋ	10	10	t	20	10
			d	20	10
			f	20	10
			v	20	10
			θ	20	10
			s	20	10
			k	20	10
			l	20	0
			r	20	10
			tʃ	20	9
			dʒ	20	10
			z	20	6
			ʃ	20	9
			g	20	10
	Total = 50 % Incorrect = 0	Total = 50		Total = 320 % Incorrect = 55	Total = 144

Analysis sheet for (+) and (−) continuant contrasts					
(+) Continuant feature			(−) Continuant feature		
Phoneme in which feature is present	Number of possible occurrences	Number of correct occurrences	Phoneme in which feature is present	Number of possible occurrences	Number of correct occurrences
f	20	0	p	20	10
v	20	0	b	20	10
θ	20	0	t	20	10
s	20	0	d	20	10
z	20	0	k	20	10
l	20	0	m	20	20
r	20	10	n	20	20
ʃ	20	1	tʃ	20	9
			dʒ	20	10
			g	20	10
			ŋ	10	10
% Incorrect = 93	Total = 160	Total = 11	% Incorrect = 38.6	Total = 210	Total = 129

Analysis sheet for (+) and (−) strident contrasts

(+) Strident feature			(−) Strident feature		
Phoneme in which feature is present	Number of possible occurrences	Number of correct occurrences	Phoneme in which feature is present	Number of possible occurrences	Number of correct occurrences
f	20	0	p	20	10
v	20	0	b	20	10
s	20	0	t	20	10
tʃ	20	8	d	20	10
dʒ	20	0	θ	20	10
z	20	3	k	20	10
ʃ	20	4	m	20	20
			n	20	20
			l	20	3
			r	20	10
			g	20	10
			ŋ	10	10
	Total = 140 % Incorrect = 89.3	Total = 15		Total = 230 % Incorrect = 42.2	Total = 133

12

Distinctive Feature Summary Sheet

When analysis sheets for all features have been completed, preliminary results may be displayed on a summary sheet. A sample of a summary sheet is presented in Table 9.

Under the heading on the summary sheet is the child's name, along with any other information the examiner wants to include. Beneath the heading are two columns. In the left column, labeled "Features," are listed the features of the distinctive feature system used. The (+) and (−) aspect of each feature is listed separately. Across from each feature is listed the percentage of error for each feature aspect. This column is labeled "Per Cent Incorrect." The percentages are obtained from the analysis sheets for each feature.

The summary table allows for a quick overview of the child's distinctive feature system errors. It does not present detailed descriptions of the status of each feature within the phonemes and contexts in which it was tested. Reference to the original articulation test data is necessary to obtain detailed information. Rather, the summary sheet presents a starting point for determining the feature or features which require training.

For developing a program for training a selected feature, a detailed analysis of the child's responses to the test phonemes is required. Details for selecting the features to be trained and the context in which the training will be administered are presented in the next part.

Table 9. Distinctive feature summary sheet

Distinctive Feature Summary Sheet

Child's name ______________________________

Articulation sample ______________________________

Date ______________________________

Examiner(s) ______________________________

Features	Per Cent Incorrect
(+) vocalic	______
(−) vocalic	______
(+) consonantal	______
(−) consonantal	______
(+) high	______
(−) high	______
(+) back	______
(−) back	______
(+) low	______
(−) low	______
(+) anterior	______
(−) anterior	______
(+) coronal	______
(−) coronal	______
(+) round	______
(−) round	______
(+) tense	______
(−) tense	______
(+) voice	______
(−) voice	______
(+) continuant	______
(−) continuant	______
(+) nasal	______
(−) nasal	______
(+) strident	______
(−) strident	______

(Additional copies of this summary sheet can be found at the back of the book.)

EXERCISES

A. Complete a distinctive feature summary sheet for Child 1.

B. Complete a distinctive feature summary sheet for Child 2.

ANSWERS TO EXERCISE A, COMPLETED SUMMARY SHEET FOR CHILD 1

Distinctive Feature Summary Sheet

Child's name Child 1

Articulation sample McDonald Deep Test of Articulation

Date May 1, 1974

Examiner(s) Engmann and McReynolds

Features	Per Cent Incorrect
(+) vocalic	27
(−) vocalic	5
(+) consonantal	15
(−) consonantal	0
(+) high	47
(−) high	17
(+) back	21
(−) back	19
(+) low	0
(−) low	9
(+) anterior	14
(−) anterior	37
(+) coronal	32
(−) coronal	8
(+) round	0
(−) round	0
(+) tense	0
(−) tense	0
(+) voice	16
(−) voice	70
(+) continuant	71
(−) continuant	9
(+) nasal	0
(−) nasal	18
(+) strident	85
(−) strident	13

ANSWERS TO EXERCISE B, COMPLETED SUMMARY SHEET FOR CHILD 2

Distinctive Feature Summary Sheet

Child's name Child 2

Articulation sample McDonald Deep Test of Articulation (first 10 responses for consonants in releasing and arresting position only)

Date May 1, 1974

Examiner(s) Engmann and McReynolds

Features	Per Cent Incorrect
(+) vocalic	75
(−) vocalic	44
(+) consonantal	47
(−) consonantal	
(+) high	80
(−) high	48
(+) back	80
(−) back	48
(+) low	
(−) low	44
(+) anterior	48
(−) anterior	68
(+) coronal	51
(−) coronal	60
(+) round	
(−) round	
(+) tense	
(−) tense	
(+) voice	43
(−) voice	96
(+) continuant	93
(−) continuant	39
(+) nasal	0
(−) nasal	55
(+) strident	89
(−) strident	42

III

DEVELOPING TRAINING PROGRAMS

After a child's distinctive feature analysis is completed and the percentage of error on features is summarized, the results provide information for developing a training program. The purpose of this chapter is to provide principles that can be used in planning a distinctive feature training program.

13

Selecting a Feature for Training

Several decisions are made concerning the child's distinctive feature system. The first decision concerns selection of the feature on which the child is to receive training. Several criteria can be applied in selecting a feature to train.

1. If the error for a feature is 25 per cent or below, the feature is considered to be established in the child's repertoire. It is not necessary to consider the feature for training.
2. Features in error at the 40 to 50 per cent level may indicate one of several patterns: (a) the feature is produced consistently in some phonemes in which it is present, but not in other phonemes in which it is present; (b) the feature is well established in phonemes in either the releasing or arresting position in words, but not in both; or (c) the child is producing the feature in appropriate contexts (phonemes) occasionally, but is also producing the feature in inappropriate contexts.
3. When the error is approximately 65 per cent, the child shows a rather inconsistent production of the feature in phonemes in which it is present. It is doubtful that the feature has been acquired or is stabilized in the child's repertoire. Therefore, it should be considered for training.
4. An error percentage of 80 per cent or above on any feature indicates that the feature has not been acquired by the child. It is lacking in his repertoire and should receive high priority for training.

If a child's profile includes error percentages on the last three levels for several features, the speech pathologist must decide which feature to select for training. The rationale presented in the first part of this book provides a basis for establishing priority. Before training features which are partially established, one should provide the child with all feature contrasts he needs for learning English phonemes. Therefore, a feature or features in error at the 80 per cent level should be trained first.

When no features are in error at the 80 per cent level, the speech pathologist may select to train a feature at the 50 or 60 per cent level. Training would be directed at stabilizing the feature across phonemes in which it is lacking, establishing it in word positions in which it is not being produced, or replacing production in inappropriate contexts with appropriate contexts.

When the feature to be trained has been selected, a phoneme pair is chosen for training the feature contrast. As stated earlier, a feature cannot be trained in isolation; it must be trained in the context of a phoneme. Selection of a phoneme pair requires information about the features composing each target phoneme and the child's substitutions for each target phoneme. According to distinctive feature theory a child must acquire both the (+) and (−) aspects of each feature; that is, he must learn feature contrasts. This fact forms the first principle for developing a training program. Furthermore, the (+) and (−) contrast has to be learned in the context of phonemes. Consequently, training involves production of two phonemes representing the feature contrast. A target phoneme possessing the (+) or (−) aspect to be trained is paired with a phoneme in which the other aspect of the feature is produced. An appropriate phoneme pair enhances the (+) and (−) aspects of the feature if the phonemes differ from each other only in the feature contrast to be learned. Training involves a production response; that is, the response is an oral one. Both phonemes are articulated during training on one feature. One of the phonemes has the (+) aspect and the other the (−) aspect of the feature. Thus, specifying a phoneme pair for feature training necessitates knowledge of the features composing a child's substitutions as well as those composing the target phonemes.

Training contexts are chosen on the basis of the child's articulation in response to the test phoneme. Each substitution for each test phoneme containing the feature to be trained is examined. Features composing them are compared and the number of features by which they differ are noted. If one of the substitutions differs from one of the target phonemes only on the feature contrast to be acquired, and the substitution is a consistent and stable one, the two phonemes may form the training context for the feature contrast.

For example, assume that a child has the (+) continuancy feature in error in 80 per cent of his productions. It is the feature selected for training. The (+) continuancy feature is present in 11 phonemes. For 8 of them the child produces substitutions consisting of phonemes which contain the (−) continuancy feature, or he omits them. He lacks (+) continuancy in /r/, /l/, /θ/, /ð/, /s/, /z/, /ʃ/, and /ʒ/. Any one of these phonemes could be selected for training the (+) continuancy feature since they all contain (+) continuancy. However, they may not all be equally suitable. Selection is determined by the phonemes on the articulation test. Thus, an examination of his substitutions for each of these test phonemes may reveal that he produces /w/ when he is tested on the /r/ and /l/. He omits the /θ/ and /ð/ in some contexts while the /h/, /t/, /d/, and /tʃ/ are produced as substitutions for them in other contexts. He omits /ʒ/ on the test and he substitutes /tʃ/ or /t/ when tested on the /s/, /z/, and /ʃ/. Keeping in mind the purpose of the training, teaching the child to produce (+) continuancy makes it desirable to select a target phoneme which differs from the child's substitution only on the contrast he is to acquire. Neither the /r/ nor the /l/ is suitable as a target phoneme to be contrasted with his /w/ substitution. Each differs from /w/ on at least seven features. Using the /w/ as a contrast for /r/ or /l/ in the hope of training (+) and (−) continuancy presents the possibility that this contrast would be obscured by all the other feature contrasts between the two phonemes. Although /θ/ and /ð/ present possible target phonemes to be contrasted with either the /t/ or /d/ because they differ only on (+) and (−) continuancy, they would not be the most appropriate sounds to teach. The child substitutes other phonemes for /θ/ and /ð/ besides /t/ and /d/. Because of the variety of substitutions it would be better to look for other phonemes which might present a more stable pattern of error. For /s/, /z/, and /ʃ/ the child produces either /t/ or /tʃ/. The /t/ differs from /s/ by two features and from the /z/ by three features. It differs from /ʃ/ by four features. Thus, using the /t/ as a comparison phoneme with either the /s/, /z/, or /ʃ/ would entail using a phoneme which contrasts with the other phoneme by more than the feature which needs to be trained. The child also produces /tʃ/ as a substitute for the /s/, /z/, and /ʃ/. Three features differentiate the /tʃ/ and /s/, and four features contrast the /z/ and /tʃ/. Therefore, pairing /tʃ/ with either the /s/ or /z/ would be pairing two phonemes which differ from each other by more than the feature to be trained. However, the /tʃ/, which is used as a substitution for /ʃ/ also, differs from /ʃ/ only on the (+) and (−) continuancy feature. It is also a stable substitution for /ʃ/. The child uses it consistently in all contexts when he is tested on /ʃ/. It would appear that the two training phonemes for teaching the child (+) and (−) continuancy should be /ʃ/ and /tʃ/.

The following exercises illustrate the procedures for selecting the appropriate feature and phoneme pair for training a feature contrast. Results from the analysis for Child 1 are used.

EXERCISES

A. Refer to the distinctive feature analysis results for Child 1 and list the features in error within the following levels:

1. 0 to 25 per cent incorrect
2. 25 to 50 per cent incorrect
3. 50 to 80 per cent incorrect
4. 80 to 100 per cent incorrect

B. Which feature should be selected for training?

C. How many phonemes are available for (+) stridency training?

D. To specify which target phoneme and corresponding substitution to select for training the (+) and (−) stridency contrast, the child's substitution for each strident phoneme is listed. Then, a comparison is made between the features composing the substitutions and the target phoneme. Finally, the number of features by which they differ is counted.

1. For Child 1, list each strident target phoneme.
2. List each corresponding substitution for each strident phoneme.
3. Specify the number of features by which the substituted phoneme differs or contrasts from the target phoneme.
4. Specify the features on which they contrast.
5. List the substitutions which differ from their target phonemes by only one feature.
6. Since the contrast to be trained is (+) and (−) stridency, which substitution and which strident target phonemes should be selected for training?

ANSWERS TO EXERCISES

A. Child 1's distinctive feature analysis shows the following levels of incorrect feature usage:

1. 0 to 25 per cent incorrect

(−) vocalic	4 per cent
(+) consonantal	15 per cent
(−) consonantal	0 per cent
(−) high	17 per cent
(+) back	21 per cent
(−) back	18 per cent
(+) low	0 per cent
(−) low	8 per cent
(+) anterior	13 per cent
(−) coronal	8 per cent
(+) round	0 per cent
(−) round	0 per cent
(+) tense	0 per cent
(−) tense	0 per cent
(+) voice	16 per cent
(−) continuant	8 per cent
(+) nasal	0 per cent
(−) nasal	17 per cent
(−) strident	13 per cent

2. 25 to 50 per cent incorrect

(+) vocalic	26 per cent
(+) high	46 per cent
(−) anterior	37 per cent
(+) coronal	31 per cent

3. 50 to 80 per cent incorrect

(−) vocalic	70 per cent
(+) continuant	71 per cent

4. 80 to 100 per cent incorrect

(+) strident	85 per cent

B. For Child 1, the feature of (+) stridency is both the highest error feature and the only feature within the 80 to 100 per cent level of incorrectness. Therefore, stridency would be the feature to choose for training.

C. Since eight phonemes are (+) strident (/f/, /v/, /s/, /z/, /ʃ/, /tʃ/, /ʒ/, /dʒ/), all are possible phonemes that should be considered for use in training stridency.

D. Substitution profile of Child 1

(+) Stridency feature

1. Target phoneme	2. Substitutions	3. Number of contrasts	4. Feature contrasts
/f/	/v/	1	Voice
	/w/	10	Consonantal, high, back, anterior, round, tense, voice, continuant nasal, strident
/v/	/b/	2	Continuant, strident
	/m/	3	Continuant, nasal, strident
/s/	/θ/	1	Strident
	/ð/	2	Strident, voice
/tʃ/	/d/	4	High, anterior, voice, strident
/dʒ/	/d/	3	High, anterior, strident
	/v/	4	Coronal, continuant, high, anterior
/z/	/d/	2	Continuant, strident
/ʃ/	/t/	4	High, anterior, strident, continuant
	/d/	5	High, anterior, continuant, strident, voice
	/g/	5	Back, coronal, voice, continuant, strident

5. The substitution of [v/f] differs in only one feature contrast, voicing. Also the substitution of [θ/s] differs in only one feature, stridency.

6. The substitution phoneme of /θ/ paired with the /s/ provides the appropriate contrast for training of the (+) strident feature.

14

Training Two Features Simultaneously

Because of the error patterns presented by some children, training one feature contrast at a time may be precluded. In other words, the child's articulation test may show that all substitutions differ from their target phonemes by at least two feature contrasts. In addition, the level of error may be the same for several features. Choosing to train (+) stridency for Child 1 presented no problem; only stridency occurred at the 80 per cent incorrect production level. Other children, however, may have more than one feature in error within that level. Such patterns sometimes make it necessary to select phoneme pairs which differ from each other on two feature contrasts. It may be more effective for these children to receive simultaneous training on the two feature contrasts on which they have a high percentage of error. Accordingly, a training program for a child with any two features, for example, continuancy and stridency, in error at the 80 per cent level can be developed. Two phonemes differing from each other in both feature contrasts would be sought. As in one-feature training, however, the phonemes should differ from each other only on the two features to be acquired. Identical principles apply in selecting phoneme pairs for two-feature training as in selecting phonemes for one-feature training. When two features are to be trained simultaneously, careful examination is required of all the features in the child's substitutions and test phonemes.

It is not possible to anticipate all feature error patterns which children with articulation errors may present. Nor is it possible to specify procedures for developing programs for all combinations of feature errors. Although similar error patterns are found among children, each child's pattern has aspects which may be peculiar to his own repertoire. In an analysis of a child's feature errors a speech pathologist should take into account the variables mentioned. This book does not offer specific programs for all possible error patterns. It offers principles of distinctive feature acquisition with the hope that they can be used by speech pathologists for developing their own procedures for individual children's feature error patterns.

Additional exercises are presented for the distinctive feature analysis of articulation errors of Child 2. They will demonstrate application of the principles to developing a training program when more than one feature contrast is to be trained simultaneously.

EXERCISES

A. List the distinctive features which are in error within the following levels for Child 2:

1. 0 to 25 per cent incorrect
2. 25 to 50 per cent incorrect
3. 50 to 80 per cent incorrect
4. 80 to 100 per cent incorrect

B. List the features which should be considered for training.

C. To decide which feature or features to train first and in what phoneme context to train the feature, list (a) each phoneme for the features of (−) voice, (+) strident and (+) continuant respectively; (b) each corresponding substitution; (c) the number of features by which the substitution phoneme differs from the target phoneme; and (d) the features on which they contrast.

D. Examining Child 2's substitution profile shows that only one of the feature contrasts could be trained alone. Which feature is this? List the reasons why the other two features cannot be trained alone.

E. For Child 2, training a single feature contrast may not be as effective as training two features simultaneously. His substitutions show that it might be possible to train either the features of (−) voice and (+) continuant together in one phoneme pair or to train (+) continuant and (+) strident simultaneously in one phoneme pair. List the phoneme pairs that could be used. Then, show why only one pair from each of the two feature contrasts would be appropriate for training two contrasts simultaneously.

F. What additional information should be considered in deciding whether to train voicing and continuancy or continuancy and stridency for Child 2?

ANSWERS TO EXERCISES

A. The distinctive feature analysis showed the following error profiles for Child 2:

1. 0 to 25 per cent incorrect

(+) nasal	0 per cent

2. 25 to 50 per cent incorrect

(−) continuant	39 per cent
(−) strident	42 per cent
(+) voice	43 per cent
(−) vocalic	44 per cent
(−) low	44 per cent
(+) consonantal	47 per cent
(−) high	48 per cent
(−) back	48 per cent
(+) anterior	48 per cent

3. 50 to 80 per cent incorrect

(+) coronal	51 per cent
(−) nasal	55 per cent
(−) coronal	60 per cent
(−) anterior	68 per cent
(+) vocalic	75 per cent

4. 80 to 100 per cent incorrect

(+) high	80 per cent
(+) back	80 per cent
(+) strident	89 per cent
(+) continuant	93 per cent
(−) voice	96 per cent

B. For Child 2, five distinctive features. (+) high, (+) back, (−) voice, (+) continuant, and (+) strident were incorrect at an 80 to 100 per cent level. Therefore, all five could be considered for training. It is possible to train one feature at a time, or it might be decided to train more than one feature at a time. Since this child has a high error rate on five features, it might be more efficient to consider selecting a phoneme pair which would provide a contrast on two of the features which have a high percentage of error.

C. Substitution profile of Child 2

(+) High feature

Target phoneme	Substitutions	Number of contrasts	Feature contrasts
/k/	/d/	5	High, back, anterior, coronal, voice
/tʃ/	/dʒ/	1	Voice
	/d/	4	High, anterior, voice, strident
/dʒ/	/d/	3	High, anterior, strident
/ʃ/	/dʒ/	2	Voice, continuant
	/t/	4	High, anterior, continuant, strident
	/d/	5	High, anterior, continuant, strident, voice
/g/	/d/	4	High, back, anterior, coronal
/ŋ/	None		

(+) Back feature

Target phoneme	Substitutions	Number of contrasts	Feature contrasts
/k/	/d/	5	High, back, anterior, coronal, voice
/g/	/d/	4	High, back, anterior, coronal
/ŋ/	None		

(−) Voice feature

Target phoneme	Substitutions	Number of contrasts	Feature contrasts
/p/	/b/	1	Voice
/t/	/d/	1	Voice
/f/	/b/	3	Voice, continuant, strident
/θ/	/d/	2	Voice, continuant
/s/	/d/	3	Voice, continuant, strident
/k/	/d/	5	High, back, anterior, coronal, voice
/h/	None		
/tʃ/	/dʒ/	1	Voice
	/d/	4	High, anterior, voice, strident
/ʃ/	/dʒ/	2	Voice, continuant
	/t/	5	High, low, anterior, continuant, strident
	/d/	6	High, low, anterior, continuant, strident, voice

(+) Strident feature

Target phoneme	Substitutions	Number of contrasts	Feature contrasts
/f/	/b/	3	Voice, continuant, strident
/v/	/b/	2	Continuant, strident
/s/	/d/	3	Voice, continuant, strident
/tʃ/	/dʒ/	1	Voice
	/d/	4	High, anterior, voice, strident
/dʒ/	/d/	3	High, anterior, strident
/z/	/dʒ/	3	High, anterior, continuant
	/d/	2	Continuant, strident
/ʃ/	/dʒ/	2	Voice, continuant
	/t/	5	High, low, anterior, continuant, strident
	/d/	6	High, low, anterior, continuant, strident, voice

(+) Continuant feature

Target phoneme	Substitutions	Number of contrasts	Feature contrasts
/f/	/b/	3	Voice, continuant, strident
/v/	/b/	2	Continuant, strident
/θ/	/d/	2	Voice, continuant
/s/	/d/	3	Voice, continuant, strident
/z/	/dʒ/	3	High, anterior, continuant
	/d/	2	Continuant, strident
/l/	/n/	3	Vocalic, continuant, nasal
/r/	/w/	11	Voice, continuant, high, back, coronal, round, tense, vocalic, continuant, nasal, strident
/h/	None		
/ʃ/	/dʒ/	2	Voice, continuant
	/t/	4	High, anterior, continuant, strident
	/d/	5	High, anterior, continuant, strident, voice

D. Only the (+) and (−) voicing contrast could be trained in the context of a phoneme pair differing in just the one feature. The child consistently substituted [b/p] and [d/t]. Either pair could be used for training. The substitution of [dʒ/tʃ] is too inconsistent to be considered for training.

The substitution profiles of Child 2 for (+) high and (+) back shows neither feature appropriate for training purposes. All of the substitutions for the (+) high and (+) back phonemes are phonemes which differ in more feature contrasts than just (+) and (−) high or (+) and (−) back. Most of the substituted phonemes differed from the target phonemes by four and five features. Because so many feature differences are present, choosing to train (+) high or (+) back first for Child 2 would not be recommended.

The child's substitutions for the (+) strident phonemes are also phonemes which differ in more than just the stridency contrast. The child does not use any substitutions in which only (+) stridency is changed to (−) stridency. In (+) continuancy, similar patterns are present. The child's (−) continuant substitutions for (+) continuant phonemes include other feature changes.

E. To train the feature contrasts of (−) voicing and (+) continuancy together, it is possible to use two phoneme pairs: [d/θ] and [dʒ/ʃ]. Examining the substitution pattern of Child 2 shows that /dʒ/ was substituted for /ʃ/ on only 3 out of 20 items. This would not be considered a consistent and stable substitution pattern. His substitution of [d/θ], however, shows a much more consistent pattern. All of his substitutions for /θ/ consisted of productions of /d/. Therefore, using the [d/θ] phoneme pair to provide the two contrasts of voicing and continuancy should provide the most effective training.

Instead of training the voicing and continuancy contrast simultaneously, it is possible to train the strident and continuant contrast together in the context of one phoneme pair. Looking at the distinctive feature results for Child 2, two phoneme pairs should be considered for training: [b/v] and [d/z]. Both of these phoneme pairs differ only in the strident and continuant contrast. Examining Child 2's substitution pattern shows that the [d/z] pair would not be selected for training the two contrasts. When /z/ was tested, Child 2 substituted /dʒ/ three times and /d/ three times. His substitution of /d/ was therefore inconsistent. However, the phoneme pair [b/v] showed a consistent pattern of production. Therefore, if the two features selected for training were (+) stridency and (+) continuancy in the context of one phoneme pair, the most efficient pair would be the [b/v].

F. A final decision concerning whether to train the voicing and continuancy contrast or the continuancy and stridency contrast would evaluate the number of phonemes affected by each of these feature errors. Training should be directed toward features in which the greatest number of phonemes are in error because such training would likely effect the most change. If the number of phonemes in error is approximately equal for both feature contrasts, then either one of them could be chosen for training.

15

Distinctive Feature Training Program

After a distinctive feature analysis has been completed and an appropriate phoneme pair has been selected, procedures for training a feature contrast are developed. A program for training distinctive features was designed for the study reported in Part I (McReynolds and Bennett, 1972). It has been used in other studies to train children with distinctive feature errors. Each procedure in the program has not been experimentally evaluated. When possible, however, the procedures were based on research. In this chapter, the program is described for clinicians interested in details of the procedures. A word of caution is in order. Since the program was designed for research purposes, it probably should not be adopted in all details for clinical use. It is offered primarily so that some of the principles on which the program is founded can be used by clinicians in designing their own training procedures. Individuals are encouraged to introduce modifications that will increase efficiency of training.

The description of the program is divided into several sections. First, definitions of the antecedent events, responses, and consequent events are presented. Second, each procedure in the program is described. The program is explained sequentially from the initial to the terminal step. Finally, the distinctive feature analysis for Child 1 is used to demonstrate each step in the program.

ANTECEDENT EVENTS

Two kinds of stimuli are included in the antecedent events: a pair of nonsense pictures and a pair of verbal nonsense syllables. The pictures are black geometric line drawings on white posterboard. The nonsense syllables may be either CV or VC syllables, depending on the phase of training. The consonant in one syllable consists of a phoneme containing the (+) aspect of a feature. The consonant in the other syllable contains the (−) aspect of the same feature. Four vowels may be used in the syllables: they are /a/, /i/, /æ/, and /u/. The vowel to be used is determined by the training phase in effect.

Each picture in a pair represents one member in a pair of nonsense syllables. The verbal stimulus accompanying the visual stimulus may be either "Say ________," in which the blank is filled with a nonsense syllable, or "What's this?" when one of the nonsense pictures is presented. The verbal stimulus is selected in accordance with the training phase in effect.

RESPONSE DEFINITION

As in many other articulation training programs, the child progresses from an imitative response to a spontaneous response in the course of training. Initially, when the clinician holds up one of the cards and says, "Say _______," the child imitates the nonsense syllables in the presence of the picture. A correct response in this phase of training is correct imitation of the nonsense syllable, or an approximation, as judged by the clinician. If approximations are accepted initially, the clinician changes criteria gradually until the response is a correct imitation of the model presented by the clinician. After the child correctly imitates the nonsense syllable, training is shifted to spontaneous production. The child produces the nonsense syllable when the clinician holds up the card and asks, "What's this?"

CONSEQUENT EVENTS

Two consequent events are used for correct responses throughout training. They consist of tokens and verbal praise (*e.g.*, "Good," "Fine," "That's right"). No consequent events are administered for incorrect responses. Tokens include marbles and plastic chips. Immediately after a correct response a marble is dropped into a plastic container. They accumulate in the container and are counted by the child and clinician at the end of each set of 20 trials during a session. If the child has earned enough marbles to reach criterion, he exchanges them for one plastic chip. A total of six plastic chips can be earned by the child in one session if he meets the criterion on six sets of 20 trials (120 trials). A plastic chip is worth one point in the reinforcer store. The toys and candy range in price from one penny to two dollars. If he wishes, a child may accumulate (save) chips until he has enough to purchase one of the more expensive toys.

Both the marbles and the verbal praise presentations change in frequency as training progresses. In the initial stages of imitation training the clinician presents a marble and praises each correct response. In other words, an FR 1 or Crf schedule is in effect. As criterion is reached, the schedule is changed to an intermittent one.

The intermittent schedule is an FR 3 (Fixed Ratio 3). The child is required to produce 3 consecutive correct responses before a marble is dropped into the container. Six marbles are needed to earn a plastic chip (the criterion remains 18 correct out of 20 responses). In the final phase of training, verbal praise is removed, but the FR 3 schedule for marbles remains in effect until terminal criterion is reached and the child is ready for generalization testing.

PRETRAINING

Before training is initiated, the child is introduced to the token system by receiving training on familiar items. He is presented with two pictures he can identify and asked to point to one named by the clinician. A pointing response is used to eliminate the possibility of reinforcing incorrect verbal responses. When 18 of the 20 marbles are accumulated, the child receives a chip and exchanges it at the token store. The schedule of reinforcement, an FR 1 schedule, is the same as the one used in the initial steps of the training program.

Several sets of trials may be presented in pretraining to acquaint the child with all contingencies. On the first, the child may receive a chip and be immediately taken to the store. On the second set, some difficult items are inserted and the child may not accumulate 18 marbles; therefore, he would not receive a plastic chip. On the third set he might earn another chip.

SESSIONS

As noted, each training session consists of 120 trials. They are presented in sets of 20 trials each; therefore, a child is presented with six sets of 20 trials per session. At the end of each set the marbles are counted, and if the child has earned a sufficient number, he is given a plastic chip. The marbles are removed from the container and the next set of 20 trials is initiated with an empty marble container.

Table 10 contains a copy of the data sheet used to record the responses during each session. The columns correspond to the six sets of 20 trials that comprise a session. After every trial the clinician records whether the response was correct or incorrect. A vertical line "|" indicates a correct response and a horizontal line "–" indicates an incorrect response. At the completion of each set of 20 trials, the correct responses are added and the total converted to a per cent correct score. Space on the sheet is provided for an observer's score. Tabulating the data after each set is essential for knowing when criterion is reached and when a plastic chip is given.

CRITERION LEVEL

Criterion must be reached at several points during the program. Criterion is specified to assure that the response is stable before a child progresses to the next step and before generalization is tested. For each 20 trial set the criterion is 18 correct responses out of 20 trials, or 90 per cent correct performance. Obtaining a plastic chip is contingent on the child having 18 marbles in the container at the end of 20 trials. Shifting from one step of the program to another is contingent on achieving 18 correct responses out of 20 trials on *three* consecutive 20-trial sets. That is, the child has to have 54 correct responses on 60 trials, and only 2 incorrect responses are allowed in each 20-trial set within the 60 trials. Shifting from one reinforcement schedule to the next is contingent on reaching a similar criterion level. For example, a child is shifted to FR 3 only after attaining 18 correct responses out of 20 trials on three 20-trial sets on the FR 1 schedule.

Emphasis is placed on testing generalization of the trained feature to other contexts. Therefore, training is structured to provide opportunities to test generalization at different levels of response acquisition.

Criterion levels are established and reinforcement schedules changed partly because generalization testing is considered important. Stringent criteria assure that the trained response is stable in the child's repertoire before transfer is tested. An intermittent reinforcement schedule is introduced for this purpose also. It shows that the response is well established in the child's repertoire.

An intermittent schedule may also serve as a framework for generalization testing during a training session. By definition, of course, generalization cannot be measured while the clinician provides consequent events for responses. If a child receives feedback on the adequacy of his response, he is being trained, not tested. Testing explores if a trained response transfers to untrained contexts when the child receives no information about the correctness of the response. For this reason, generalization is usually tested only after training has been completed. That is, it is tested aside from the training procedure. It is possible, however, to test generalization during training if a child is on an intermittent schedule of reinforcement. For example, on an FR 3 schedule a child is accustomed to producing two responses without receiving any information

Table 10. Data sheet for recording responses during a training session

Child ______________________

Phase ______________________

Date ______________________

	Set I	Set II	Set III	Set IV	Set V	Set VI
Trial 1						
Trial 2						
Trial 3						
Trial 4						
Trial 5						
Trial 6						
Trial 7						
Trial 8						
Trial 9						
Trial 10						
Trial 11						
Trial 12						
Trial 13						
Trial 14						
Trial 15						
Trial 16						
Trial 17						
Trial 18						
Trial 19						
Trial 20						
Per cent correct						
Clinician						
Observer						

about them. He only receives feedback after the third response. On training items 1 and 2 no consequent event is presented. Therefore, if a generalization item is inserted in trial 1 or 2, no feedback needs to be presented; the child doesn't receive it during training on those items either. One generalization item (one probe item) can replace one of the unreinforced training items (trials) without interfering with the training procedure or the child's behavior. Similar items can be inserted in trials 4 and 5, 7 and 8, and so on.

In the program presented in this chapter, transfer is tested in two contexts on the McDonald Deep Test. First, transfer of the trained phoneme from nonsense syllables to words is tested with the phoneme in both releasing and arresting positions. This testing is used to evaluate whether a phoneme trained in a nonsense syllable transfers to words. Second, transfer of the feature to other phonemes in which the feature had been in error is evaluated. These are phonemes which had been misarticulated on the McDonald Deep Test and received no treatment. All releasing and arresting items on the McDonald Test for the particular phonemes under test are presented. Because of the experimental nature of the program, probes are presented whenever a child reaches criterion in each step of the program. This results in numerous tests. It is probably unnecessary to probe as often in a clinical situation.

PROCEDURES

The program may start with training on an isolated phoneme for one feature aspect acquisition, or two phonemes in nonsense syllables for immediate feature contrast acquisition. (Actually, in producing an isolated phoneme, it becomes a syllable for most sounds.) In the experimental program, isolated phoneme training precedes contrast training. In either case, the sequence moves from imitation to spontaneous production.

Imitation

In isolated phoneme training the clinician presents the phoneme in association with one of the nonsense pictures. That is, the consonant containing the feature aspect the child needs to acquire is trained alone first. The clinician holds up the picture and when the child attends, says "Say _______." If the response is judged correct by the clinician, a marble is dropped into a container placed close to the child. If the response is judged incorrect, the clinician puts the picture down, waits approximately 10 seconds, then initiates a new trial.

At the end of 20 trials the marbles are counted and the child is told whether he has earned enough to receive a chip. The token transaction is completed and a new set of 20 trials is started. When six sets of 20 trials have been completed, the session is terminated. Tokens earned by the child are counted and a trip to the store follows.

Criterion levels are not in effect until the child is imitating the model correctly. In other words, no approximations can be occurring for criterion performance. When a level of 18 correct responses out of 20 trials in three consecutive sets is reached, the schedule is changed to an FR 3 schedule. The child is told he now needs 6 marbles, instead of 18, to earn a token. Although the number of marbles changes, the criterion does not. It remains 18/20. After reaching criterion on FR 3 imitation, training is shifted to spontaneous production.

Spontaneous Production

Because of the shift from imitation to spontaneous production, a continuous reinforcement schedule (FR 1) is reintroduced in the initial stages. The clinician holds up the picture and asks, "What's this?" For each correct response the child is presented with a marble, but verbal praise is no longer given. As before, incorrect responses are not consequated.

Criterion performance on the FR 1 schedule is two sets of 20 trials each at a 90 per cent (18/20) level of correctness. When criterion is reached, training is shifted to the FR 3 schedule. Criterion for FR 3 performance is three sets of 20 trials at 90 per cent correct.

When criterion is reached in FR 3 spontaneous production training, the child is presented with the generalization test items. Usually, the marbles, marble container, and training stimuli are removed from the table. The pictures in the McDonald Deep Test are presented for all phonemes containing the feature being trained, and the child's responses are transcribed on the test sheet.

The words containing the trained phoneme in releasing and arresting positions are presented first. Next, the other phonemes containing the feature are presented. These phonemes have been selected on the basis of the child's performance on the original articulation test. If the feature is in error in approximately 65 per cent or more of the items, then the phoneme is included in the test.

If the child shows transfer to 80 per cent of the items in all the test phonemes, training for that feature is terminated. This is a very uncommon occurrence. Seldom does generalization occur before contrast training is initiated. Therefore, as usually happens, the child evidences no generalization, or very limited generalization after isolated phoneme training. If generalization does not occur, the child progresses to the next step in the program, training in the feature contrast.

Feature Contrast Training

Training now exposes the child to both the (+) and (−) aspects of the feature. Both phonemes representing the feature contrast are trained. If the child has received the preceding isolated phoneme training, the clinician introduces both nonsense syllables and both nonsense pictures in this step.

In one of the nonsense syllables the consonant has the (+) aspect of the feature, and the consonant in the other nonsense syllable has the (−) aspect. Usually, the first vowel context in which the consonants are presented is the /a/.

During contrast training, the clinician holds up one of the pictures, models the nonsense syllable associated with the picture, and waits for the child to imitate the model. In the next trial, the same picture and nonsense syllable may be presented, or the clinician may pick up the other picture and model the second syllable for imitation. In other words, each 20-trial set is now divided into 10 presentations of each of the two pictures and are presented in random order.

Procedures for training the two syllables are identical to the procedures used for training the isolated phoneme. Training proceeds from imitation to spontaneous production, and from an FR 1 to an FR 3 schedule of reinforcement. The only difference is that the child now has to produce two different consonants correctly when presented with their pictures. When criterion is reached on FR 3 spontaneous production, the generalization items are presented again.

Training is continued in this manner. Additional nonsense syllables are trained until 80 per cent feature generalization occurs. Usually the vowels /a/, /i/, /æ/, and /u/ are used to form the nonsense syllables.

The contrast pairs are trained in the context of each vowel in the initial position first, followed by training in the final position. If the feature has not generalized after the four vowel contexts have been trained in both positions, a second phoneme pair is selected for training the same feature. The same procedures are followed in training the second pair as were followed for training the first pair.

To demonstrate the procedures, the training program for Child 1 is presented in Table 11.

Table 11. Distinctive feature training procedures for Child 1 (+) stridency feature

	Phase	Response mode	Reinforcement schedule	Criteria
Phase 1.	Phoneme representing (+) or (–) aspect of feature in error trained in isolation			
Training context 1	Phoneme representing error feature trained in isolation			
	Step 1. Stimulus is /s/	1. Imitative–"Say /s/"	1. FR 1–Verbal praise and tokens	1. 90 per cent correct on three consecutive sets of 20 trials each
	Step 2. Stimulus is /s/	2. Imitative–"Say /s/"	2. FR 3–Verbal praise and tokens	2. 90 per cent correct on three consecutive sets of 20 trials each
	Step 3. Stimulus is /s/	3. Spontaneous–"What's this?"	3. FR 1–Tokens only	3. 90 per cent correct on two consecutive sets of 20 trials each
	Step 4. Stimulus is /s/	4. Spontaneous–"What's this?"	4. FR 3–Tokens only	4. 90 per cent correct on three consecutive sets of 20 trials each
Probe	Probe test for all strident phonemes: /s/, /f/, /v/, /z/, /tʃ/, /dʒ/, /ʃ/	Spontaneous response to the McDonald Deep Test items for all seven strident phonemes	No reinforcement	Train an additional training context until 80 per cent generalization of stridency occurs to the seven strident phonemes
Phase 2.	Phoneme pair representing (+) and (–) feature contrast trained in arresting position of four nonsense syllables.			
Training context 1	Phoneme pair trained in context of low back vowel			
	Step 1. Stimuli are /as/–/aθ/	1. Imitative–"Say /as/–/aθ/"	1. FR 1–Verbal praise and tokens	1. 90 per cent correct on three consecutive sets of 20 trials each
	Step 2. Stimuli are /as/–/aθ/	2. Imitative–"Say /as/–/aθ/"	2. FR 3–Verbal praise and tokens	2. 90 per cent correct on three consecutive sets of 20 trials each
	Step 3. Stimuli are /as/–/aθ/	3. Spontaneous–"What's this?"	3. FR 1–Tokens only	3. 90 per cent correct on two consecutive sets of 20 trials each
	Step 4. Stimuli are /as/–/aθ/	4. Spontaneous–"What's this?"	4. FR 3–Tokens only	4. 90 per cent correct on three consecutive sets of 20 trials each
Probe	Probe test for all strident phonemes: /s/, /t/, /v/, /z/, /tʃ/, /dʒ/, /ʃ/	Spontaneous response to the McDonald Deep Test items for all seven strident phonemes	No reinforcement	Train an additional training context until 80 per cent generalization of stridency occurs to the seven strident phonemes

	Phase	Response mode	Reinforcement schedule	Criteria
Training context 2	Phoneme pair trained in context of high front vowel			
	Step 1. Stimuli are /is/–/iθ/	1. Imitative–"Say /is/–/iθ/"	1. FR 1–Verbal praise and tokens	1. 90 per cent correct on three consecutive sets of 20 trials each
	Step 2. Stimuli are /is/–/iθ/	2. Imitative–"Say /is/–/iθ/"	2. FR 3–Verbal praise and tokens	2. 90 per cent correct on three consecutive sets of 20 trials each
	Step 3. Stimuli are /is/–/iθ/	3. Spontaneous–"What's this?"	3. FR 1–Tokens only	3. 90 per cent correct on two consecutive sets of 20 trials each
	Step 4. Stimuli are /is/–/iθ/	4. Spontaneous–"What's this?"	4. FR 3–Tokens only	4. 90 per cent correct on three consecutive sets of 20 trials each
Probe	Probe test for all strident phonemes: /s/, /f/, /v/, /z/, /tʃ/, /dʒ/, /ʃ/	Spontaneous response to the McDonald Deep Test items for all seven strident phonemes	No reinforcement	Train an additional training context until 80 per cent generalization of stridency occurs to the seven strident phonemes
Training context 3	Phoneme pair trained in context of low front vowel			
	Step 1. Stimuli are /æs/ and /æθ/	1. Imitative–"Say /æs/ and /æθ/"	1. FR 1–Verbal praise and tokens	1. 90 per cent correct on three consecutive sets of 20 trials each
	Step 2. Stimuli are /æs/ and /æθ/	2. Imitative–"Say /æs/ and /æθ/"	2. FR 3–Verbal praise and tokens	2. 90 per cent correct on three consecutive sets of 20 trials each
	Step 3. Stimuli are /æs/ and /æθ/	3. Spontaneous–"What's this?"	3. FR 1–Tokens only	3. 90 per cent correct on two consecutive sets of 20 trials each
	Step 4. Stimuli are /æs/ and /æθ/	4. Spontaneous–"What's this?"	4. FR 3–Tokens only	4. 90 per cent correct on three consecutive sets of 20 trials each
Probe	Probe test for all strident phonemes: /s/, /f/, /v/, /z/, /tʃ/, /dʒ/, /ʃ/	Spontaneous response to the McDonald Deep Test items for all seven strident phonemes	No reinforcement	Train an additional training context until 80 per cent generalization of stridency occurs to the seven strident phonemes
Training context 4	Phoneme pair trained in context of high back vowel			
	Step 1. Stimuli are /us/–/uθ/	1. Imitative–"Say /us/–/uθ/"	1. FR 1–Verbal praise and tokens	1. 90 per cent correct on three consecutive sets of 20 trials each
	Step 2. Stimuli are /us/–/uθ/	2. Imitative–"Say /us/–/uθ/"	2. FR 3–Verbal praise and tokens	2. 90 per cent correct on three consecutive sets of 20 trials each
	Step 3. Stimili are /us/–/uθ/	3. Spontaneous–"What's this?"	3. FR 1–Tokens only	3. 90 per cent correct on two consecutive sets of 20 trials each
	Step 4. Stimuli are /us/–/uθ/	4. Spontaneous–"What's this?"	4. FR 3–Tokens only	4. 90 per cent correct on three consecutive sets of 20 trials each

	Phase	Response mode	Reinforcement schedule	Criteria
Probe	Probe test for all strident phonemes: /s/, /f/, /v/, /z/, /tʃ/, /dʒ/, /ʃ/	Spontaneous response to the McDonald Deep Test items for all seven strident phonemes	No reinforcement	Train an additional training context until 80 per cent generalization of stridency occurs to the seven strident phonemes
Phase 3.	Phoneme pair representing (+) and (–) feature contrast trained in releasing position of nonsense syllables			
Training context 1	Phoneme pair trained in context of low back vowel			
	Step 1. Stimuli are /sa/ and /θa/	1. Imitative–"Say /sa/–/θa/"	1. FR 1–Verbal praise and tokens	1. 90 per cent correct on three consecutive sets of 20 trials each
	Step 2. Stimuli are /sa/ and /θa/	2. Imitative–"Say /sa/–/θa/"	2. FR 3–Verbal praise and tokens	2. 90 per cent correct on three consecutive sets of 20 trials each
	Step 3. Stimuli are /sa/ and /θa/	3. Spontaneous–"What's this?"	3. FR 1–Tokens only	3. 90 per cent correct on two consecutive sets of 20 trials each
	Step 4. Stimuli are /sa/ and /θa/	4. Spontaneous–"What's this?"	4. FR 3–Tokens only	4. 90 per cent correct on three consecutive sets of 20 trials each
Probe	Probe test for all strident phonemes: /s/, /t/, /v/, /z/, /tʃ/, /dʒ/, /ʃ/	Spontaneous response to the McDonald Deep Test items for all seven strident phonemes	No reinforcement	Train an additional training context until 80 per cent generalization of stridency occurs to the seven strident phonemes
Training context 2	Phoneme pair trained in context of high front vowel			
	Step 1. Stimuli are /si/ and /θi/	1. Imitative–"Say /si/–/θi/"	1. FR 1–Verbal praise and tokens	1. 90 per cent correct on three consecutive sets of 20 trials each
	Step 2. Stimuli are /si/ and /θi/	2. Imitative–"Say /si/–/θi/"	2. FR 3–Verbal praise and tokens	2. 90 per cent correct on three consecutive sets of 20 trials each
	Step 3. Stimuli are /si/ and /θi/	3. Spontaneous–"What's this?"	3. FR 1–Tokens only	3. 90 per cent correct on two consecutive sets of 20 trials each
	Step 4. Stimuli are /si/ and /θi/	4. Spontaneous–"What's this?"	4. FR 3–Tokens only	4. 90 per cent correct on three consecutive sets of 20 trials each
Probe	Probe test for all strident phonemes: /s/, /t/, /v/, /z/, /tʃ/, /dʒ/, /ʃ/	Spontaneous response to the McDonald Deep Test items for all seven strident phonemes	No reinforcement	Repeat training procedures using a different phoneme pair representing stridency contrast

Training context 3	**Phoneme pair trained in context of low front vowel**			
	Step 1. Stimuli are /sæ/ and /θæ/	1. Imitative–"Say /sæ/–/θæ/"	1. FR 1–Verbal praise and tokens	1. 90 per cent correct on three consecutive sets of 20 trials each
	Step 2. Stimuli are /sæ/ and /θæ/	2. Imitative–"Say /sæ/–/θæ/"	2. FR 3–Verbal praise and tokens	2. 90 per cent correct on three consecutive sets of 20 trials each
	Step 3. Stimuli are /sæ/ and /θæ/	3. Spontaneous–"What's this?"	3. FR 1–Tokens only	3. 90 per cent correct on two consecutive sets of 20 trials each
	Step 4. Stimuli are /sæ/ and /θæ/	4. Spontaneous–"What's this?"	4. FR 3–Tokens only	4. 90 per cent correct on three consecutive sets of 20 trials each
Probe	Probe test for all strident phonemes: /s/, /t/, /v/, /z/, /tʃ/, /dʒ/, /ʃ/	Spontaneous response to the McDonald Deep Test items for all seven strident phonemes	No reinforcement	Repeat training procedures using a different phoneme pair representing stridency contrast
Training context 4	Phoneme pair trained in context of high back vowel			
	Step 1. Stimuli are /su/–/θu/	1. Imitative–"Say /su/–/θu/"	1. FR 1–Verbal praise and tokens	1. 90 per cent correct on three consecutive sets of 20 trials each
	Step 2. Stimuli are /su/–/θu/	2. Imitative–"Say /su/–/θu/"	2. FR 3–Verbal praise and tokens	2. 90 per cent correct on three consecutive sets of 20 trials each
	Step 3. Stimuli are /su/–/θu/	3. Spontaneous–"What's this?"	3. FR 1–Tokens only	3. 90 per cent correct on two consecutive sets of 20 trials each
	Step 4. Stimuli are /su/–/θu/	4. Spontaneous–"What's this?"	4. FR 3–Tokens only	4. 90 per cent correct on three consecutive sets of 20 trials each
Probe	Probe test for all strident phonemes: /s/, /f/, /v/, /z/, /tʃ/, /dʒ/, /ʃ/	Spontaneous response to the McDonald Deep Test items for all seven strident phonemes	No reinforcement	Repeat training procedures using a different phoneme pair representing stridency contrast

16

Summary to Part III

A distinctive feature analysis is time-consuming in comparison to some other articulation assessment procedures. It is an in-depth examination of a child's articulation errors, the systematic nature of these errors, and the relationship between his phonological system and the adult's. For many clinicians the time element may be the factor determining whether a distinctive feature analysis should be conducted. The time involved in completing an analysis should be weighed against the hours spent in assessing and training when an analysis is not completed. Each clinician will make his or her own decision in the context of individual caseloads and schedules.

Naturally, a distinctive feature analysis should be completed primarily when children have several sounds in error. If a child misarticulates fewer than four phonemes, a distinctive feature analysis probably is not useful, unless detailed, context-specific rules are desired. For this purpose, procedures similar to those developed by Compton might be applied in addition to the broader analysis presented in this book.

A clinician may not wish to use the feature set proposed by Chomsky and Halle and applied in this book. If not, others are available. Turton (1973), for example, suggests using a place and manner set in a feature analysis. A feature system has been proposed by Singh and his colleagues (1972), as well as by Walsh (1974). The Fisher-Logemann Test (1971) employs a place and manner analysis. Several other feature systems could be adopted for this purpose (*e.g.*, Wickelgren, 1966; Peters, 1963; and Miller and Nicely, 1971). Among these, with the exception of the Fisher-Logemann Test, the systems appear to be in the proposal stage still. That is to say, no empirical data have been published concerning their use in analysis of children's misarticulations.

Some of the feature systems employ narrow transcription. Such detail allows notation of distortions. In effect, nondistinctive features can be recorded. A detailed, narrow transcription might lead to development of more efficient and effective training programs for children. Clearly, the procedures are justified if they contribute information leading to better training procedures. When narrow transcription is proposed, speech pathologists should ask themselves the same questions they ask when a distinctive feature analysis is proposed. What will it contribute to the therapy program? Would it change the procedures proposed in this book for phoneme selection and for training? How would these be changed? If changes result, they should be evaluated in light of the terminal goals of the program. If they function to increase efficiency of training, they should be adopted. It is well to keep in mind that all procedures, including those proposed in this text, can and should be evaluated empirically by speech pathologists. A desire to provide the best possible service dictates that clinicians do so. They should welcome the opportunity to consider alternatives, to test all of them, and institute changes on the basis of data obtained in their clinical environments. Throughout the book clinicians have been encouraged to conduct their own objective investigations of all proposed evaluation and training procedures. This admonition is reiterated once more.

Regardless of the system used, a response analysis allows a careful, in-depth examination of what the child is producing, and the rules or patterns which account for his errors. Any analysis that compares the dimensions of what the child is producing with the dimensions of what he should be producing is an evaluation based on the child's behavior. Rather than using external criteria for developing a training program, therapy is derived directly from the child's responses. Since it is *this* behavior that needs to be modified, it would appear an excellent place to begin assessment.

It is hoped that clinicians, whenever appropriate, will use the analysis and training procedures from this book in conjunction with other procedures that have been shown to be effective. In this way, both the child and the clinician may accomplish articulation modification in less time and with less effort.

IV REFERENCES

Albright, R. and Albright, J., Application of descriptive linguistics to child language. *Journal of Speech and Hearing Research,* 1, 257-261 (1958).

Applegate, J., Phonological rules of a subdialect of English. *Word,* 17, 186-193 (1961).

Bar-Adon, A. and Leopold, W., *Child Language: A Book of Readings.* Englewood Cliffs, New Jersey: Prentice-Hall (1971).

Berko, J. and Brown, R., Psycholinguistic research methods. In P. H. Mussen (Ed.), *Handbook of Research Methods in Child Development.* New York: Wiley (1960).

Cairns, C. and Williams, F., Language. In F. D. Minifie, T. J. Hixon, and F. Williams (Eds.), *Normal Aspects of Speech, Hearing, and Language.* Englewood Cliffs, New Jersey: Prentice-Hall (1973).

Chomsky, N. and Halle, M., *The Sound Pattern of English.* New York: Harper and Row (1968).

Compton, A., Generative studies of children's phonological disorders. *Journal of Speech and Hearing Disorders,* 35, 315-339 (1970).

Crocker, J., A phonological model of children's articulation competence. *Journal of Speech and Hearing Disorders,* 34, 203-213 (1969).

Delattre, P., From acoustic cues to distinctive features. *Phonetica,* 18, 198-230 (1968).

Elbert, M., Shelton, R. L., and Arndt, W. B., A task for the evaluation of articulation change: 1, Development of methodology. *Journal of Speech and Hearing Research,* 10, 281-288 (1967).

Fant, C., Distinctive features and phonetic dimensions. In G. E. Perren and J. L. Trim (Eds.), *Application of Linguistics.* New York: Cambridge University Press (1971).

Farquhar, M., Prognostic value of imitative and auditory discrimination tests. *Journal of Speech and Hearing Disorders,* 26, 342-347 (1961).

Ferguson, C. and Slobin, D. (Eds.), *Studies in Child Language Development.* New York: Holt, Rinehart and Winston (1973).

Fisher, H. B. and Logemann, J. A., *The Fisher-Logemann Test of Articulation Competence.* New York: Houghton Mifflin (1971).

Graham, L. and House, A., Phonological oppositions in children: a perceptual study. *The Journal of the Acoustical Society of America,* 49, 559-566 (1971).

Haas, W., Phonological analysis of a case of dyslalia. *Journal of Speech and Hearing Disorders,* 28, 239-246 (1963).

Jakobson, R., *Studies on Child Language and Aphasia.* The Hague: Mouton (1971).

Jakobson, R., Fant, C., and Halle, M., *Preliminaries to Speech Analysis.* Cambridge, Massachusetts: MIT Press (1952).

Jakobson, R. and Halle, M., *Fundamentals of Language.* The Hague: Mouton (1956).

Lieberman, A., Cooper, F., Shankweiler, D., and Studdert-Kennedy, M., Perception of the speech code. *Psycholinguistic Review,* 74, 431-461 (1967).

MacNeilage, P., Motor control of serial ordering of speech. *Psychological Review,* 77, 182-196 (1970).

McDonald, E., *Articulation Testing and Treatment: A Sensory-Motor Approach.* Pittsburgh: Stanwix House (1964).

McDonald, E., *A Deep Test of Articulation: Picture Form.* Pittsburgh: Stanwix House (1964).

McLean, J. E., Extending stimulus control of phoneme articulation by operant techniques. In F. L. Girardeau and J. D. Spradlin (Eds.), *A Functional Analysis Approach to Speech and Language,* ASHA Monograph 14. Washington, D.C.: American Speech and Hearing Association (1970).

McReynolds, L. and Bennett, S., Distinctive feature generalization in articulation training. *Journal of Speech and Hearing Disorders,* 37, 462-470 (1972).

McReynolds, L. and Huston, K., A distinctive feature analysis of children's misarticulations. *Journal of Speech and Hearing Disorders,* 36, 155-166 (1971).

Menyuk, P., The role of distinctive features in children's acquisition of phonology. *Journal of Speech and Hearing Research,* 11, 138-146 (1968).

Miller, G. and Nicely, P., An analysis of perceptual confusions among some English consonants. *Journal of the Acoustical Society of America,* 27, 338-352 (1955).

Peters, R., Dimensions of perception for consonants. *Journal of the Acoustical Society of America,* 35, 1985-1989 (1963).

Peterson, C. and Shoup, J., A physiological theory of phonetics. *Journal of Speech and Hearing Research,* 9, 5-67 (1966).

Poole, I. Genetic development in articulation of consonant sounds in speech. *Elementary English,* II, 159-161 (1934).

Postal, P., *Aspects of Phonological Theory.* New York: Harper and Row (1968).

Saporta, S., Frequency of consonant clusters. *Language,* 31, 25-30 (1955).

Shelton, R. L., Elbert, M., and Arndt, W. B., A task for evaluation of articulation change: II. Comparison of task scores during baseline and lesson series testing. *Journal of Speech and Hearing Research,* 10, 578-585 (1967).

Singh, S., Perceptual similarities and minimal phonemic differences. *Journal of Speech and Hearing Research,* 14, 113-124 (1971).

Singh, S., *Distinctive Features: Theory and Validation,* Baltimore: University Park Press (1975).

Singh, S. and Becker, G., A comparison of four feature systems using data from three psychophysical methods. *Journal of Speech and Hearing Research,* 15, 821-829 (1972).

Singh, S. and Black, J., Study of twenty-six intervocalic consonants spoken and recognized by four language groups. *Journal of the Acoustical Society of America,* 39, 372-387 (1966).

Singh, S., Woods, D., and Becker, C., Perceptual structure of twenty-two prevocalic English consonants. *Journal of the Acoustical Society of America,* 52, 1698-1713 (1972).

Snow, K. and Milisen, R., The influence of oral versus pictorial representation upon articulation testing results. *Journal of Speech and Hearing Disorders, Monograph Supplement 4,* 29-36 (1954).

Spriestersbach, D. and Curtis, J., Misarticulation and discrimination of speech sounds. *Quarterly Journal of Speech,* 37, 483-491 (1951).

Templin, M. Certain language skills in children, their development and interrelationships. *Institute of Child Welfare, Monograph Series No. 26.* Minneapolis: University of Minnesota Press (1957).

Turton, L. J., Diagnostic implications of articulation testing. In W. D. Wolfe and D. J. Goulding (Eds.), *Articulation and Learning,* Springfield, Illinois: Charles C Thomas (1973).

Walsh, H., On certain practical inadequacies of distinctive feature systems. *Journal of Speech and Hearing Disorders,* 39, 32-43 (1974).

Wellman, B., Case, I., Mengert, I., and Bradbury, D., Speech sounds of young children. *University of Iowa Studies in Child Welfare,* 5, No. 2 (1931).

Wickelgren, W., Distinctive features and errors in short term memory for English consonants. *Journal of the Acoustical Society of America,* 39, 388-398 (1966).

Wilson, R., A criticism of distinctive features. *Journal of Linguistics,* 2, 195-206 (1966).

Winitz, H., *Articulatory Acquisition and Behavior.* New York: Appleton-Century-Crofts (1969).

Wood, K., Measurement of progress in the correction of articulatory speech defects. *Journal of Speech and Hearing Disorders,* 14, 171-174 (1949).

Index

ADDITIONAL WORKSHEET
from McReynolds & Engmann:
Distinctive Feature Analysis of Misarticulations
University Park Press   Baltimore

Distinctive feature analysis worksheet

Test phoneme ___________

	Test phoneme and number of times correct	Phonemes substituted and number of occurrences	Number of omissions	Number of times features used correctly
	____ ____	____ ____ ____ ____ ____ ____	____	____ ____
Vocalic				
Consonantal				
High				
Back				
Low				
Anterior				
Coronal				
Round				
Tense				
Voice				
Continuant				
Nasal				
Strident				

ADDITIONAL WORKSHEET
from McReynolds & Engmann:
Distinctive Feature Analysis of Misarticulations
University Park Press Baltimore

Distinctive feature analysis worksheet

Test phoneme ___________

	Test phoneme and number of times correct	Phonemes substituted and number of occurrences	Number of omissions	Number of times features used correctly
	____ ____	____ ____ ____ ____ ____ ____	____	____ ____
Vocalic				
Consonantal				
High				
Back				
Low				
Anterior				
Coronal				
Round				
Tense				
Voice				
Continuant				
Nasal				
Strident				

ADDITIONAL WORKSHEET
from McReynolds & Engmann:
Distinctive Feature Analysis of Misarticulations
University Park Press Baltimore

Distinctive feature analysis worksheet

Test phoneme ____________

	Test phoneme and number of times correct	Phonemes substituted and number of occurrences	Number of omissions	Number of times features used correctly
	_____ _____	_____ _____ _____ _____ _____ _____	_____	_____ _____
Vocalic				
Consonantal				
High				
Back				
Low				
Anterior				
Coronal				
Round				
Tense				
Voice				
Continuant				
Nasal				
Strident				

ADDITIONAL WORKSHEET
from McReynolds & Engmann:
Distinctive Feature Analysis of Misarticulations
University Park Press Baltimore

Distinctive feature analysis worksheet

Test phoneme ________

	Test phoneme and number of times correct	Phonemes substituted and number of occurrences	Number of omissions	Number of times features used correctly
	____ ____	____ ____ ____ ____ ____ ____	____	____ ____
Vocalic				
Consonantal				
High				
Back				
Low				
Anterior				
Coronal				
Round				
Tense				
Voice				
Continuant				
Nasal				
Strident				

ADDITIONAL WORKSHEET
from McReynolds & Engmann:
Distinctive Feature Analysis of Misarticulations
University Park Press Baltimore

Distinctive feature analysis worksheet

Test phoneme ________

	Test phoneme and number of times correct	Phonemes substituted and number of occurrences	Number of omissions	Number of times features used correctly
	____ ____	____ ____ ____ ____ ____ ____	____	____ ____
Vocalic				
Consonantal				
High				
Back				
Low				
Anterior				
Coronal				
Round				
Tense				
Voice				
Continuant				
Nasal				
Strident				

ADDITIONAL WORKSHEET
from McReynolds & Engmann:
Distinctive Feature Analysis of Misarticulations
University Park Press Baltimore

Distinctive feature analysis worksheet

Test phoneme ________

	Test phoneme and number of times correct	Phonemes substituted and number of occurrences	Number of omissions	Number of times features used correctly
	____ ____	____ ____ ____ ____ ____ ____	____	____ ____
Vocalic				
Consonantal				
High				
Back				
Low				
Anterior				
Coronal				
Round				
Tense				
Voice				
Continuant				
Nasal				
Strident				

ADDITIONAL WORKSHEET
from McReynolds & Engmann:
Distinctive Feature Analysis of Misarticulations
University Park Press Baltimore

Distinctive feature analysis worksheet

Test phoneme ______

	Test phoneme and number of times correct	Phonemes substituted and number of occurrences	Number of omissions	Number of times features used correctly
	____ ____	____ ____ ____ ____ ____ ____	____	____ ____
Vocalic				
Consonantal				
High				
Back				
Low				
Anterior				
Coronal				
Round				
Tense				
Voice				
Continuant				
Nasal				
Strident				

ADDITIONAL WORKSHEET
from McReynolds & Engmann:
Distinctive Feature Analysis of Misarticulations
University Park Press Baltimore

Distinctive feature analysis worksheet

Test phoneme ____________

	Test phoneme and number of times correct	Phonemes substituted and number of occurrences	Number of omissions	Number of times features used correctly
	_____ _____	_____ _____ _____ _____ _____ _____	_____	_____ _____
Vocalic				
Consonantal				
High				
Back				
Low				
Anterior				
Coronal				
Round				
Tense				
Voice				
Continuant				
Nasal				
Strident				

ADDITIONAL WORKSHEET
from McReynolds & Engmann:
Distinctive Feature Analysis of Misarticulations
University Park Press Baltimore

Distinctive feature analysis worksheet

Test phoneme ______

	Test phoneme and number of times correct	Phonemes substituted and number of occurrences	Number of omissions	Number of times features used correctly
	____ ____	____ ____ ____ ____ ____ ____	____	____ ____
Vocalic				
Consonantal				
High				
Back				
Low				
Anterior				
Coronal				
Round				
Tense				
Voice				
Continuant				
Nasal				
Strident				

ADDITIONAL WORKSHEET
from McReynolds & Engmann:
Distinctive Feature Analysis of Misarticulations
University Park Press   Baltimore

Distinctive feature analysis worksheet

Test phoneme ________

	Test phoneme and number of times correct	Phonemes substituted and number of occurrences	Number of omissions	Number of times features used correctly
	____ ____	____ ____ ____ ____ ____ ____	____	____ ____
Vocalic				
Consonantal				
High				
Back				
Low				
Anterior				
Coronal				
Round				
Tense				
Voice				
Continuant				
Nasal				
Strident				

ADDITIONAL WORKSHEET
from McReynolds & Engmann:
Distinctive Feature Analysis of Misarticulations
University Park Press Baltimore

Distinctive feature analysis worksheet

Test phoneme ______

	Test phoneme and number of times correct	Phonemes substituted and number of occurrences	Number of omissions	Number of times features used correctly
	___ ___	___ ___ ___ ___ ___ ___	___	___ ___
Vocalic				
Consonantal				
High				
Back				
Low				
Anterior				
Coronal				
Round				
Tense				
Voice				
Continuant				
Nasal				
Strident				

ADDITIONAL WORKSHEET
from McReynolds & Engmann:
Distinctive Feature Analysis of Misarticulations
University Park Press Baltimore

Distinctive feature analysis worksheet

Test phoneme ____________

	Test phoneme and number of times correct	Phonemes substituted and number of occurrences	Number of omissions	Number of times features used correctly
	____ ____	____ ____ ____ ____ ____ ____	____	____ ____
Vocalic				
Consonantal				
High				
Back				
Low				
Anterior				
Coronal				
Round				
Tense				
Voice				
Continuant				
Nasal				
Strident				

ADDITIONAL WORKSHEET
from McReynolds & Engmann:
Distinctive Feature Analysis of Misarticulations
University Park Press Baltimore

Distinctive feature analysis sheet

Analysis sheet for (+) and (−) ____________ contrasts

(+) ____________ Feature			(−) ____________ Feature		
Phoneme in which feature is present	Number of possible occurrences	Number of correct occurrences	Phoneme in which feature is present	Number of possible occurrences	Number of correct occurrences
	Total = ______	Total = ______		Total = ______	Total = ______
	% Incorrect = ______			% Incorrect = ______	

ADDITIONAL WORKSHEET
from McReynolds & Engmann:
Distinctive Feature Analysis of Misarticulations
University Park Press Baltimore

Distinctive feature analysis sheet

Analysis sheet for (+) and (−) ______________ contrasts					
(+) ______________ Feature			(−) ______________ Feature		
Phoneme in which feature is present	Number of possible occurrences	Number of correct occurrences	Phoneme in which feature is present	Number of possible occurrences	Number of correct occurrences
	Total = _______	Total = _______		Total = _______	Total = _______
	% Incorrect = _______			% Incorrect = _______	

ADDITIONAL WORKSHEET
from McReynolds & Engmann:
Distinctive Feature Analysis of Misarticulations
University Park Press Baltimore

Distinctive feature analysis sheet

Analysis sheet for (+) and (−) ____________ contrasts					
(+) ____________ Feature			(−) ____________ Feature		
Phoneme in which feature is present	Number of possible occurrences	Number of correct occurrences	Phoneme in which feature is present	Number of possible occurrences	Number of correct occurrences
	Total = ______	Total = ______		Total = ______	Total = ______
	% Incorrect = ______			% Incorrect = ______	

ADDITIONAL WORKSHEET
from McReynolds & Engmann:
Distinctive Feature Analysis of Misarticulations
University Park Press Baltimore

Distinctive feature analysis sheet

Analysis sheet for (+) and (−) _____________ contrasts

(+) _____________ Feature			(−) _____________ Feature		
Phoneme in which feature is present	Number of possible occurrences	Number of correct occurrences	Phoneme in which feature is present	Number of possible occurrences	Number of correct occurrences
	Total = _______	Total = _______		Total = _______	Total = _______
	% Incorrect = _______			% Incorrect = _______	

ADDITIONAL WORKSHEET
from McReynolds & Engmann:
Distinctive Feature Analysis of Misarticulations
University Park Press Baltimore

Distinctive feature analysis sheet

Analysis sheet for (+) and (−) ____________ contrasts

(+) ____________ Feature			(−) ____________ Feature		
Phoneme in which feature is present	Number of possible occurrences	Number of correct occurrences	Phoneme in which feature is present	Number of possible occurrences	Number of correct occurrences
	Total = ______	Total = ______		Total = ______	Total = ______
	% Incorrect = ______			% Incorrect = ______	

ADDITIONAL WORKSHEET
from McReynolds & Engmann:
Distinctive Feature Analysis of Misarticulations
University Park Press Baltimore

Distinctive feature analysis sheet

Analysis sheet for (+) and (−) ____________ contrasts

(+) ____________ Feature			(−) ____________ Feature		
Phoneme in which feature is present	Number of possible occurrences	Number of correct occurrences	Phoneme in which feature is present	Number of possible occurrences	Number of correct occurrences
	Total = ______	Total = ______		Total = ______	Total = ______
	% Incorrect = ______			% Incorrect = ______	

ADDITIONAL WORKSHEET
from McReynolds & Engmann:
Distinctive Feature Analysis of Misarticulations
University Park Press Baltimore

Distinctive feature analysis sheet

Analysis sheet for (+) and (−) ____________ contrasts					
(+) ____________ Feature			(−) ____________ Feature		
Phoneme in which feature is present	Number of possible occurrences	Number of correct occurrences	Phoneme in which feature is present	Number of possible occurrences	Number of correct occurrences
	Total = ______	Total = ______		Total = ______	Total = ______
% Incorrect = ______			% Incorrect = ______		

ADDITIONAL WORKSHEET
from McReynolds & Engmann:
Distinctive Feature Analysis of Misarticulations
University Park Press Baltimore

Distinctive feature analysis sheet

Analysis sheet for (+) and (−) ______________ contrasts

(+) ______________ Feature			(−) ______________ Feature		
Phoneme in which feature is present	Number of possible occurrences	Number of correct occurrences	Phoneme in which feature is present	Number of possible occurrences	Number of correct occurrences
	Total = _______	Total = _______		Total = _______	Total = _______
	% Incorrect = _______			% Incorrect = _______	

ADDITIONAL WORKSHEET
from McReynolds & Engmann:
Distinctive Feature Analysis of Misarticulations
University Park Press Baltimore

Distinctive feature analysis sheet

Analysis sheet for (+) and (−) ______ contrasts					
(+) ______ Feature			(−) ______ Feature		
Phoneme in which feature is present	Number of possible occurrences	Number of correct occurrences	Phoneme in which feature is present	Number of possible occurrences	Number of correct occurrences
	Total = ______	Total = ______		Total = ______	Total = ______
	% Incorrect = ______			% Incorrect = ______	

ADDITIONAL WORKSHEET
from McReynolds & Engmann:
Distinctive Feature Analysis of Misarticulations
University Park Press Baltimore

Distinctive feature analysis sheet

Analysis sheet for (+) and (−) ______________ contrasts

(+) ______________ Feature			(−) ______________ Feature		
Phoneme in which feature is present	Number of possible occurrences	Number of correct occurrences	Phoneme in which feature is present	Number of possible occurrences	Number of correct occurrences
	Total = _______	Total = _______		Total = _______	Total = _______
	% Incorrect = _______			% Incorrect = _______	

ADDITIONAL WORKSHEET
from McReynolds & Engmann:
Distinctive Feature Analysis of Misarticulations
University Park Press Baltimore

Distinctive feature analysis sheet

Analysis sheet for (+) and (−) ______________ contrasts

(+) ______________ Feature			(−) ______________ Feature		
Phoneme in which feature is present	Number of possible occurrences	Number of correct occurrences	Phoneme in which feature is present	Number of possible occurrences	Number of correct occurrences
	Total = _______	Total = _______		Total = _______	Total = _______
% Incorrect = _______			% Incorrect = _______		

ADDITIONAL WORKSHEET
from McReynolds & Engmann:
Distinctive Feature Analysis of Misarticulations
University Park Press Baltimore

Distinctive feature analysis sheet

Analysis sheet for (+) and (−) ____________ contrasts

(+) ____________ Feature			(−) ____________ Feature		
Phoneme in which feature is present	Number of possible occurrences	Number of correct occurrences	Phoneme in which feature is present	Number of possible occurrences	Number of correct occurrences
	Total = _______	Total = _______		Total = _______	Total = _______
	% Incorrect = _______			% Incorrect = _______	

ADDITIONAL WORKSHEET
from McReynolds & Engmann:
Distinctive Feature Analysis of Misarticulations
University Park Press Baltimore

Distinctive feature summary sheet

Distinctive Feature Summary Sheet

Child's name ____________________

Articulation sample ____________________

Date ____________________

Examiner(s) ____________________

Features	Per Cent Incorrect
(+) vocalic	______
(−) vocalic	______
(+) consonantal	______
(−) consonantal	______
(+) high	______
(−) high	______
(+) back	______
(−) back	______
(+) low	______
(−) low	______
(+) anterior	______
(−) anterior	______
(+) coronal	______
(−) coronal	______
(+) round	______
(−) round	______
(+) tense	______
(−) tense	______
(+) voice	______
(−) voice	______
(+) continuant	______
(−) continuant	______
(+) nasal	______
(−) nasal	______
(+) strident	______
(−) strident	______

ADDITIONAL WORKSHEET
from McReynolds & Engmann:
Distinctive Feature Analysis of Misarticulations
University Park Press Baltimore

Distinctive feature summary sheet

Distinctive Feature Summary Sheet

Child's name ______________________________

Articulation sample ______________________________

Date ______________________________

Examiner(s) ______________________________

Features	Per Cent Incorrect
(+) vocalic	________
(−) vocalic	________
(+) consonantal	________
(−) consonantal	________
(+) high	________
(−) high	________
(+) back	________
(−) back	________
(+) low	________
(−) low	________
(+) anterior	________
(−) anterior	________
(+) coronal	________
(−) coronal	________
(+) round	________
(−) round	________
(+) tense	________
(−) tense	________
(+) voice	________
(−) voice	________
(+) continuant	________
(−) continuant	________
(+) nasal	________
(−) nasal	________
(+) strident	________
(−) strident	________